617. SHE
026

D1330544

Surgical Emergencies
in Clinical Practice

Iqbal Shergill • Manit Arya
Tahwinder Upile • Neehar Arya
Prokar Dasgupta
Editors

Surgical Emergencies in Clinical Practice

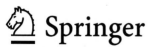 Springer

Editors

Iqbal Shergill, B.Sc.(Hons),
MRCS FRCS (Urol),
Department of Urology
Wrexham Maelor Hospital
Betsi Cadwaladr University
Health Board
Wrexham
Wales
UK

Manit Arya, MBChB, M.D.,
FRCS(Glasgow), FRCS(Urol)
Department of Urological
Oncology
University College Hospital
London and
Department of Experimental
Medicine
The Barts Cancer Institute
London
UK

Tahwinder Upile, B.Sc.(hons),
M.Sc., M.S., M.D., FRCS (Gen
Surg), FRCS (OTO), FRCS
(ORL-HNS), DFFP, FHEA,
MRCGP,
ENT Department
Barnet & Chase Farm
Hospital/UCLH
London
UK

Neehar Arya M.B.B.S., B.Sc.
(Hons), FRCSEd., FCEM,
Department of Emergency
Medicine
Sturgeon Community Hospital
St. Albert
Alberta
Canada

Prokar Dasgupta, M.Sc. (Urol),
M.D., DLS, FRCS (Urol),
FEBU, MRC
Department of Urology and
Department of Surgery
Centre for Transplantation
NIHR Biomedical Research Centre
Kings College London, Guy's Campus
London
UK

ISBN 978-1-4471-2875-5   ISBN 978-1-4471-2876-2 (eBook)
DOI 10.1007/978-1-4471-2876-2
Springer London Heidelberg New York Dordrecht

Library of Congress Control Number: 2012945469

© Springer-Verlag London 2013
This work is subject to copyright. All rights are reserved by the Publisher,
whether the whole or part of the material is concerned, specifically the rights
of translation, reprinting, reuse of illustrations, recitation, broadcasting, repro-
duction on microfilms or in any other physical way, and transmission or
information storage and retrieval, electronic adaptation, computer software,
or by similar or dissimilar methodology now known or hereafter developed.
Exempted from this legal reservation are brief excerpts in connection with
reviews or scholarly analysis or material supplied specifically for the purpose
of being entered and executed on a computer system, for exclusive use by
the purchaser of the work. Duplication of this publication or parts thereof is per-
mitted only under the provisions of the Copyright Law of the Publisher's location, in its current version, and permission for use must always be obtained
from Springer. Permissions for use may be obtained through RightsLink at
the Copyright Clearance Center. Violations are liable to prosecution under the
respective Copyright Law.
The use of general descriptive names, registered names, trademarks, service
marks, etc. in this publication does not imply, even in the absence of a specific
statement, that such names are exempt from the relevant protective laws and
regulations and therefore free for general use.
While the advice and information in this book are believed to be true and accurate at the date of publication, neither the authors nor the editors nor the publisher can accept any legal responsibility for any errors or omissions that may be
made. The publisher makes no warranty, express or implied, with respect to the
material contained herein.

Printed on acid-free paper

Springer is part of Springer Science+Business Media (www.springer.com)

To all those with surgical spirit about them!

Foreword

With the introduction of new post-graduate training, virtually all doctors will be exposed to some form of surgical training prior to specialization. Many of these doctors will have little exposure to certain surgical emergencies in medical school. Thus, they may unnecessarily refer to a senior doctor when not needed or catastrophically neglect a patient needing urgent surgical opinion.

This book has been written for exam preparation and for daily clinical practice, so that all surgical trainees may benefit from the combined experience of the team who wrote the book. Each chapter includes key features of history and examination that enables the understanding of what is required in day-to-day clinical practice. The principles of acute management are described, allowing the reader to understand the importance of emergency management and the implications of not applying the key principles. This will hopefully prevent some of the mistakes that we all would have made in managing such patients when we were juniors.

We feel that this book will be a valuable tool for all junior doctors and medical students, and it will also be of interest to nurse practitioners, general practitioners, and allied health professionals managing these patients. We sincerely hope it will be of clinical benefit to the patients that we treat on a daily basis.

Contents

Contributors

Shafiq Ahmed, M.B.B.S., M.S., DNB (Urology)
Department of Urology, Christian Medical College and
Hospital, Ludhiana, Punjab, India

Department of Genitourinary Surgery, Christian Medical
College and Hospital, Ludhiana, Punjab, India

Tan Arulampalam, M.B.B.S., M.D., FRCS
Department of Laparoscopic and Colorectal Surgery,
Iceni Centre, Colchester Hospital University NHS
Foundation Trust, Essex, UK

Manit Arya, MBChB, M.D., FRCS (Glasgow), FRCS (Urol)
Department of Urological Oncology, University College
Hospital, London

Department of Experimental
Medicine, The Barts Cancer Institute, London, UK

Neehar Arya, M.B.B.S., B.Sc. (Hons), FRCSEd., FCEM
Department of Emergency Medicine, Sturgeon Community
Hospital, St. Albert, Alberta, Canada

Alan Askari, MBChB, MRCS
Department of Orthopaedics, Colchester Hospital
University Foundation NHS Trust, Essex, UK

Great Western Hospitals NHS Foundation Trust,
Swindon, UK

David Choi, M.A., MBChB, FRCS, Ph.D.
Department of Neurosurgery, Institute of Neurology
and Neurosurgery, University College London, London, UK
Department of Neurosurgery, The National Hospital
for Neurology and Neurosurgery, London, UK

Alun H. Davies, M.A., DM, FRCS, FHEA, FEBVS, FACPh
Department of Vascular Surgery, Charing Cross Hospital,
Imperial College Healthcare NHS Trust,
London, UK

Faculty of Medicine, Charing Cross Hospital,
Imperial College School of Medicine,
London, UK

**Prokar Dasgupta, M.Sc. (Urol), M.D., DLS, FRCS (Urol),
FEBU, MRC**
Department of Urology and Department of Surgery,
Centre for Transplantation, NIHR Biomedical Research
Centre, Kings College London, London, UK

Susan Drinkwater
Department of Vascular Surgery, Royal Preston Hospital,
Lancashire, UK

Timothy Hammett, M.A., M.B.B.S., MRCS
Centre for Spinal Studies and Surgery,
Queens Medical Centre, Nottingham, UK

Alan W. Hewitt, M.A., FRCS (SN)
Department of Spine Surgery, James Cook University
Hospital, Middlesbrough, Teeside, UK

Colin Hopper, FRCS, M.D.
Head and Neck Unit, University College London Hospitals,
London, UK

Waseem Jerjes, B.Sc. (hons), Ph.D., M.Sc., B.D.S., M.B.B.S.
Department of ENT, Barnet and Chase Farm Hospitals,
Enfield, Greater London, UK

Jaspal Mahil, B.Sc. (hons), MRCGP, DFFP
Department of ENT, Barnet and Chase Farm Hospitals,
Enfield, Greater London, UK

Kim Mammen, M.S., MCh, DNB, FRCS, FACS
Department of Urology, Christian Medical College
and Hospital, Ludhiana, Punjab, India

Rohan J. Mammen, M.B.B.S.
Department of Urology, Christian Medical College
and Hospital, Ludhiana, Punjab, India

**Jitendra Mangwani, M.B.B.S. (GOLD MEDAL), M.S.
(ORTH), FRCS (TR & ORTH)**
Department of Trauma and Orthopaedics,
University Hospitals of Leicester, Leicester Royal Infirmary,
Leicester, UK

Pari-Naz Mohanna, M.B.B.S., B.Sc., M.D., FRCS (plast)
Department of Plastic and Reconstructive Surgery,
Guy's and St. Thomas' NHS Foundation Trust,
London, UK

Narain Moorjani, MBChB, MRCS, M.D., FRCS (C-Th)
Department of Cardiothoracic Surgery,
Papworth Hospital, University of Cambridge,
Cambridge, UK

Vikas Pandey, M.D., FRCS
Regional Vascular Unit, St. Mary's Hospital, Imperial
College Healthcare NHS Trust, London, UK

N. Patel, FRCS
Head and Neck Unit, Department of ENT, Southampton
University Hospitals, Southampton, UK

Nikhil Pawa, M.D., LLM, M.Sc., MRCS
Department of General Surgery, Watford General Hospital,
Hertfordshire, UK

Krishna Penumetcha, B.Sc. (hons), MRCGP, DFFP
Department of ENT, Barnet and Chase Farm Hospitals,
Enfield, Greater London, UK

Heman E.S. Prasad, M.B.B.S., M.S. (Surgery)
Department of Urology, Christian Medical College
and Hospital, Ludhiana, Punjab, India

Samer Saour, MB, BCh, BAO, MRCS, M.Sc.
Department of Plastic and Reconstructive Surgery,
Guys and St Thomas' NHS Foundation Trust, London, UK

Iqbal Shergill, B.Sc. (Hons), MRCS, FRCS (Urol)
Department of Urology, Wrexham Maelor Hospital,
Betsi Cadwaladr University Health Board,
Wrexham, Wales, UK

Janavikulam Thiruchelvam, FRCS, M.D.
Oral Maxillofacial Unit, Head and Neck Department,
Barnet and Chase Farm Hospitals, Greater London, UK

Matthew Thomas, M.B.B.S., MRCS
Department of Urology, Royal Liverpool and Broadgreen
University Hospitals, Liverpool, UK

Navdeep Upile, B.Sc. (hons), MRCD, DOHNS
Department of ENT, Aintree University Hospital NHS
Foundation Trust, Liverpool, UK

**Tahwinder Upile, B.Sc. (hons), M.Sc., M.S., M.D., FRCS
(Gen Surg), FRCS (OTO), FRCS (ORL-HNS), DFFP,
FHEA, MRCGP**
Department of ENT, Barnet and Chase Farm Hospitals,
Enfield, Greater London, UK

Head and Neck Unit, University College London Hospitals,
Greater London, UK

**Stephen Westaby, B.Sc., FRCS, M.S., Ph.D., FESC, FACC,
FECTS, FICA**
Department of Surgery, John Radcliffe Hospital,
Oxford, UK

Chapter 1
General Surgical Emergencies

Nikhil Pawa, Timothy Hammett, and Tan Arulampalam

Introduction

General surgery is the largest surgical subspecialty, and, as such, all junior trainees are expected to pass through general surgical placements during their rotations. In addition, many general surgical emergencies manifest themselves in patients in other surgical specialties, as well as in medical wards and in the accident and emergency setting. Hence, general surgical conditions are extremely common, and dealt with by all trainees throughout their surgical training.

Although the scope of emergencies is extremely vast, in day-to-day practice, only a few common emergencies make up the workload of an emergency "on call." Hence, in this chapter, only these common general surgical emergencies are dealt

N. Pawa, M.D., LLM, M.Sc., MRCS (✉)
Department of General Surgery, Watford General Hospital,
Hertfordshire, UK
e-mail: nikhil@pawa.me.uk

T. Hammett, M.A., M.B.B.S., MRCS
Centre for Spinal Studies and Surgery, Queens Medical Centre,
Nottingham, UK

T. Arulampalam, M.B.B.S., M.D., FRCS
Department of Laparoscopic and Colorectal Surgery,
Iceni Centre, Colchester Hospital University
NHS Foundation Trust, Essex, UK

I. Shergill et al. (eds.), *Surgical Emergencies in Clinical Practice*,   1
DOI 10.1007/978-1-4471-2876-2_1,
© Springer-Verlag London 2013

with, highlighting the key features of history and examination that will allow expeditious diagnosis, as well as allowing an understanding of the vast differential diagnoses that may coexist. Importantly, the information supplied will be useful for those in other surgical specialties, who may not have had early exposure to general surgery, to understand the important concepts and to deal appropriately with these emergencies. One of the key themes in general surgery is that emergency management involves appropriate resuscitation and medical treatment initially to try and improve patient's overall condition, in anticipation for emergency operative surgery when indicated.

Clinical Case Scenario 1: Right Iliac Fossa Pain

Case Presentation

A 16-year-old female presents to accident and emergency department with a 24-h history of worsening continuous abdominal pain, initially located in the umbilical region, then migrating to the right iliac fossa. She has been vomiting, but otherwise has no bowel or urogenital symptoms, and is otherwise fit and well, taking only the oral contraceptive pill. Her last period was 1 week previously. On examination, she is mildly febrile, with a pulse of 90 bpm, and has localized tenderness with rebound and guarding in the right lower quadrant. Her urine dipstick is negative.

Key Features of History and Examination

The relevant features of the history and examination include the following:

- Worsening, continuous abdominal pain, rather than sudden onset, indicates a progressive inflammatory process rather than a ruptured/perforated viscus. The typical symptom is of migratory pain – initially involving the visceral peritoneum, which localizes pain to the midline. Then, as the inflammation progresses, it involves the more sensitive parietal peritoneum which localizes pain to the right iliac fossa. Associated nausea and vomiting is a common finding.

- Diarrhea or constipation does not rule out appendicitis by any means, but diarrhea and rectal bleeding/mucus discharge or other gastrointestinal (GI) manifestations (ulcers/abscesses) should raise the possibility of Crohn's disease, particularly if there is a positive family history.
- All patients with abdominal pain should be asked about urinary symptoms of dysuria, frequency, and offensive urine.
- A sexual history is crucial, particularly in young patients, as both pelvic inflammatory disease and ectopic pregnancy can cause severe pain and systemic upset, and ask directly regarding sexually transmitted infections and pregnancy. *A urinary pregnancy test is mandatory in fertile females presenting with abdominal pain.* With this, a history of gynecological problems, menstrual cycle, and previous investigations should also be included.
- Examination may reveal a low-grade pyrexia and a degree of tachycardia. Tenderness should be maximal over McBurney's point (one-third of the distance from the right anterior superior iliac spine and umbilicus). Palpate for guarding and rebound tenderness. Check for Rovsing's sign – palpation in the left iliac fossa causes pain in the right iliac fossa, obturator sign-right iliac fossa pain with internal/external rotation of the flexed right hip, or psoas sign-right iliac fossa pain with extension of the right hip.
- Signs and symptoms may also vary with the position of the appendix. A retrocecal appendix (62%) can manifest as right loin or upper quadrant tenderness, with a pelvic (34%) appendix causing diarrhea and urinary symptoms.
- Hernial orifices should also be examined and external genitalia in the male.

Principles of Acute Management

The differential diagnosis is listed in Table 1.1, and, importantly, the causes that need to be ruled out first and foremost include

TABLE 1.1 Differential diagnosis of acute appendicitis

Patient group	Possible diagnoses
Young patients	Ectopic pregnancy
	Pelvic inflammatory disease
	Ruptured ovarian follicle
	Ovarian cyst torsion
	Endometriosis
	Inflammatory bowel disease
	Testicular torsion
	Gastroenteritis
	Mesenteric adenitis
	UTI
	Meckel's diverticulitis
Older patients	Diverticulitis
	Tubo-ovarian pathology
	Cecal perforation
	UTI

ectopic pregnancy (ruptured or otherwise) and testicular torsion in the younger population. Management of all patients includes establishing intravenous access and administering fluids, keeping the patient nil by mouth, administering adequate analgesia and antiemetics. In cases of sepsis or patients undergoing surgery, intravenous antibiotics should be administered. A period of observation is reasonable in borderline cases without peritoneal or septic signs. Investigations, including imaging, can be organized to aid the diagnosis.

Blood Tests

A raised white cell count (WCC) is seen in 80–85% of cases of appendicitis. Many studies advocate the use of C-reactive protein (CRP) testing to aid diagnosis.

Urinalysis

This is important to exclude urinary tract infections and pregnancy.

Ultrasound Scan

Ultrasound has a sensitivity of 81% for appendicitis. The use of this test should be reserved for when the diagnosis is uncertain, usually in women.

CT

This can be used in patients with atypical presentations including masses palpable on examination. CT is probably the most sensitive preoperative diagnostic imaging tool.

The treatment of choice for appendicitis remains an appendicectomy. This is now performed increasingly by the laparoscopic approach. A Cochrane review in 2004 reported a shorter hospital stay in patients undergoing a laparoscopic appendicectomy in comparison with open surgery together with an early return to normal activities and work [2]. Laparoscopy also gives excellent views of the pelvic organs and allows the surgeon full access to inspect the small bowel for cases of a Meckel's diverticulum and therefore useful in cases of diagnostic uncertainty.

The complications of acute appendicitis include peritonitis, perforation, appendiceal abscesses, hemorrhage, other abscesses, and intestinal obstruction. Perforation of a gangrenous appendix causes peritonitis leading to the development of intra-abdominal abscesses. Often, the patients show signs of significant shock. Abscesses must be broken down and thorough peritoneal lavage performed.

In certain cases, the perforation and abscess may be walled off by surrounding omentum and loops of bowel forming a mass. This can be confirmed by imaging and the abscess drained percutaneously. Many surgeons advocate the concept of an interval appendicectomy (6 weeks onward) to prevent any further complications and rule out any other conditions.

Discussion

Right iliac fossa pain is one of the most common presenting complaints to a general surgical take, with a variety of diagnoses. A ruptured ectopic pregnancy must be excluded in all fertile females. Acute appendicitis is a clinical diagnosis commonly developing in children and young adults. Patients can present septic and should be resuscitated aggressively. Appendicectomy remains the treatment of choice, although in cases of poor surgical candidates, nonoperative management can be attempted with variable results.

Five Key Points

1. Appendicitis is the most common surgical cause of the acute abdomen accounting for 17% of presentations.
2. The appendix is highly mobile and unpredictable in location. Signs will depend on the location of the appendix.
3. Observation is a perfectly valid reason for admission and is a valid diagnostic modality in cases of doubt. There will often be conflicting results from bloods/urine – remember this is predominantly a clinical diagnosis.
4. Exclude the major causes of abdominal pain – ectopic pregnancy, testicular torsion that can all present in a similar manner.
5. Treat appendicitis with appendicectomy unless patient is too unwell to consider operative intervention or in the case of appendicular mass.

Clinical Case Scenario 2: Right Upper Quadrant Pain

Case Presentation

A 45-year-old lady presents to the accident and emergency department in the middle of the night with severe right upper quadrant abdominal pain radiating to the back. She has vomited

TABLE 1.2 Differential diagnosis of right upper quadrant pain

Biliary colic	Cholecystitis
Acute pancreatitis	Gastritis
Gastroenteritis	Pneumonia
Myocardial infarction	Hepatitis
Peptic ulcer disease	Renal colic
Appendicitis	Hepatic abscess

approximately six times and has been feeling feverish throughout the night with a loss of appetite. Both her bowel and urinary habits have been normal. The rest of her history is unremarkable. On examination, she is pyrexial at 38.0°C with a pulse of 105 bpm. Her blood pressure and oxygen saturations are stable. Abdominal examination reveals tenderness in the right upper quadrant.

Key Features of History and Examination

The differential diagnosis of right upper quadrant pain is listed in Table 1.2. Commonly, it is a result of gallstone disease, and this may present in a number of ways. A careful history and examination can help distinguish between them.

Biliary Colic

This typically consists of intermittent episodes of right upper quadrant abdominal pain radiating to the shoulder and back. This type of pain is visceral in origin caused by distension of the gallbladder by obstruction. The onset of pain is often hours after a meal, commonly at night, and can persist for up to 24 h with associated nausea and vomiting. Examination may demonstrate some tenderness in the right upper quadrant.

Acute Cholecystitis

This is typified by constant right upper quadrant pain (parietal) lasting longer than 24 h associated with nausea/vomiting and anorexia. It is caused by impaction of a stone in Hartmann's pouch or the cystic duct which causes a sterile inflammation followed by secondary bacterial infection. Examination often reveals a fever, tachycardia with marked tenderness in the right upper quadrant, accentuated during inspiration (Murphy's sign). Up to 70% of people report a previous history of biliary symptoms.

Empyema of the Gallbladder

This is usually results from stone impaction obstructing the cystic duct in the presence of acute cholecystitis. This progresses to a suppurative infection filling the gallbladder with purulent material. The patient presents toxic with a swinging fever and tachycardia. Examination often reveals a palpable large tender mass in the right upper quadrant.

Choledocholithiasis

This occurs when stones migrate from the gallbladder into the bile duct (12% of cases). In some cases, the stones will pass spontaneously, in others they become impacted within the common bile duct causing obstructive jaundice (painful). Typically the urine is dark due to bilirubin with pale stools (low stercobilinogen) with mild jaundice.

Ascending Cholangitis

This is usually caused by bacterial infection in the presence of partial or complete obstruction of the biliary system. It is commonly associated with Gram-negative bacteria (*E. Coli*). Patients present with a combination of right upper quadrant pain, rigors, and jaundice (Charcot's triad).

Principles of Acute Management

Investigations for right upper quadrant pain usually provide a good indication of underlying diagnosis and causality.

Blood Tests

Raised inflammatory markers suggest septic complications. Liver function tests should be performed, with raised bilirubin and alkaline phosphatase (ALP) suggesting biliary obstruction or cholangitis. In cases of jaundice, a clotting screen should be performed due to underlying liver dysfunction.

US Abdomen

This should be performed on all acute presentations. It can identify 95% of gallstones and provide information on features of inflammation (thickened wall, pericholecystic fluid). It also provides information on dilatation of the biliary tree suggesting obstruction.

Endoscopic Retrograde Cholangiopancreatography

Endoscopic retrograde cholangiopancreatography (ERCP) is probably the most valuable technique for the management of obstructive jaundice. It allows visualization of stones or strictures within the biliary tree. Stones can be removed with the help of baskets, and stents can abridge strictures, and, finally, the option of sphincterotomy can be utilized, if appropriate. Cytological and histological samples can also be obtained from the pancreas and biliary tree.

Magnetic Resonance Cholangiopancreatography

This is a noninvasive study with a sensitivity of 95% for the detection of biliary obstruction. It is useful in diagnosing the cause of obstructive jaundice (ductal stones, lesions in the head of the pancreas, or cholangiocarcinoma).

In the emergency setting, up to 95% of patients with biliary colic settle with adequate analgesia and dietary restrictions (fat-free diet). Many patients that present to hospital often require strong opiates. Encouragingly, almost four out of five patients presenting with acute cholecystitis recover with good analgesia, fluid resuscitation, intravenous antibiotics, and dietary restriction.

Laparoscopic cholecystectomy is the gold standard procedure for symptomatic gallstone disease. In the UK, some centers perform this in the emergency setting following investigations, although typically patients are often discharged home, with a view to performing this electively. Patients developing empyemas of the gallbladder, who are often unfit to undergo a cholecystectomy, can be managed by a percutaneous cholecystostomy (under radiological guidance) in the emergency setting.

Discussion

Increasingly acute laparoscopic cholecystectomies are being performed for patients presenting with uncomplicated gallstone disease. This can shorten total hospital stay and be more cost effective. Generally speaking, surgery should be performed within the first 3 days of symptom onset to hospital to minimize risks.

Common bile duct stones can be managed in various ways. Commonly, an ERCP can be performed to extract the stones and perform sphincterotomy before cholecystectomy. An alternative is a one-stage procedure including exploration of the common bile duct (open or laparoscopic) at the time of cholecystectomy. The advantages of the second approach are a shorter hospital stay, and it is also more cost effective. A Cochrane review in 2006 reported no significant difference in morbidity and mortality between laparoscopic exploration of the duct and preoperative or postoperative ERCP with equally efficient stone clearance [1].

Key Points

1. Right upper quadrant pain is usually due to gallstones, which are common and in up to 12% of men and 24% of women.

2. Gallstone disease presents in various ways, and a thorough history and examination must be performed to distinguish between them.
3. An abdominal ultrasound scan should be performed to assess for the presence of stones, features of cholecystitis, and biliary tree dilatation.
4. Laparoscopic cholecystectomy is the optimum management of symptomatic gallstone disease. This can be performed as a day case procedure in healthy patients and in the acute setting with little risks.
5. Common bile duct stones can be managed by either ERCP pre/postoperatively or exploration of the duct at surgery.

Clinical Case Scenario 3: Bowel Obstruction

Case Presentation

A 65-year-old man presents with a 3-day progressive history of colicky, central abdominal pain and distension, absolute constipation, and, more recently, vomiting. On direct questioning, he admits to intermittent dark rectal blood for the last few months and has lost about a stone in weight. On examination, he is a febrile, with normal observations. His abdomen is massively distended and has no obvious scars. He is tympanic to percussion, and there is no tenderness to palpation. Rectal examination reveals an empty, collapsed rectum. Chest X-ray is normal, but abdominal radiograph demonstrates distended ascending and transverse colon with an abrupt cut-off in the sigmoid colon.

Key Features of History and Examination

This case presentation demonstrates the classic symptoms of intestinal obstruction (large bowel) – absolute constipation, colicky abdominal pain, distension, and vomiting. Distinction between large and small bowel obstruction can be made through history and examination and confirmed radiologically.

TABLE 1.3 Causes of bowel obstruction

| Small bowel obstruction | | Large bowel obstruction | |
Cause	Incidence (%)	Cause	Incidence (%)
Adhesions	70–80	Colonic tumor	65
Hernias	10–15	Miscellaneous (pseudo-obstruction)	20
Tumor	5–10	Diverticular disease	10–20
Other (Crohn's)	<5	Volvulus	5

Typically, small bowel obstruction often presents with vomiting early and less distension, while large bowel obstruction presents with distension and constipation early developing vomiting later. The causes of small and large bowel obstruction are listed in Table 1.3.

The initial history should focus on ascertaining the onset and nature of symptoms. A sudden acute onset may indicate a volvulus. The patient should be questioned regarding any recent change in bowel habit or rectal bleeding together with loss of weight or appetite. Any previous history of abdominal surgery or investigations should be noted. Small bowel obstruction commonly occurs with adhesions following previous surgery. Multiple medications slow gut transit and can cause pseudo-obstruction or true obstruction secondary to fecal impaction. Some of the most common culprits are opiates and benzodiazepines. Antipsychotic medication is also frequently implicated. Any significant family history of malignancy or diverticular disease should be noted.

On examination, patients can present pyrexial (possible infarction, perforation) and with signs of shock. The entire abdomen must be examined, checking in particular for scars, and making a thorough check of the hernia orifices (inguinal and femoral). Percussion will most likely be resonant. Tenderness or peritonitis should raise suspicion of perforation or ischemia. Auscultation would most likely reveal absent or tinkling bowel sounds. PR may reveal the collapsed, empty rectum of obstruction or be heavily fecally loaded in cases of impaction.

Principles of Acute Management

Initial investigations would include the following:

Blood Tests

These tests are performed to looking for anemia, raised inflammatory markers, and signs of dehydration. In cases where infarction or perforation is suspected clinically, an arterial blood gas is useful.

X-Rays

A plain abdominal radiograph is usually diagnostic for bowel obstruction with numerous distended loops of small bowel seen for small bowel obstruction and a proximal dilated colon with a cutoff for large bowel obstruction. In cases of an incompetent ileocecal valve, there may be some partial decompression into the small bowel. A chest film should also be performed to exclude coexisting perforation (free air under the diaphragm).

Water-Soluble Enema

This test is useful in large bowel obstruction differentiating between a pseudo-obstruction and a mechanical cause, and typically gastrografin (water-soluble contrast) is used.

CT Scan

This is usually performed to identify the cause and stage the disease in cases of malignancy, or where diagnosis is in doubt.

The initial management of small bowel obstruction includes fluid resuscitation (due to significant third space losses), restriction of oral intake (keep patient "nil by mouth"), adequate analgesia, and nasogastric decompression. A urinary catheter is also placed and hourly urine output monitored. Regular blood tests should be performed to monitor the urea and electrolytes.

Approximately 80% of cases of adhesional small bowel obstruction will settle with such conservative measures. Surgery for small bowel obstruction is indicated in the following cases: where intestinal ischemia is suspected, an irreducible hernia, failed conservative management (24–48 h), or in cases of no previous surgical history (virgin abdomen). The old adage of "never let the sun set twice on a case of small bowel obstruction" still holds true in contemporary surgical practice.

Patients should be reviewed regularly as any changes in clinical condition such as localized peritonitis or the development of an acidosis could mean impending strangulation and surgery should be planned immediately. At surgery, the cause is identified and small bowel inspected. If an infarction is present, a resection and primary anastomosis is performed. If the cause is found to be a hernia, mesh placement is often avoided if resection is necessary due to the high risk of infection.

With regard to large bowel obstruction, pseudo-obstruction is commonly managed by identifying and correcting any electrolyte abnormalities and avoiding causative drugs. Surgery is associated with a high morbidity and mortality and therefore avoided. If a volvulus is identified on radiograph (classic inverted bean), decompression is attempted by rigid sigmoidoscopy and passage of rectal tube. In certain cases, a flexible sigmoidoscopy may be necessary allowing decompression and inspection of the colon for necrosis.

In cases of tumor or diverticular stricture, resection is the preferred treatment choice. Colonic stents can be used in patients not fit for surgical resection to decompress the obstruction, and also in certain patients to plan for an elective procedure and primary anastomosis. Patients undergoing surgery should be warned about the possibility of a stoma. Surgery is usually performed open in these cases.

Right-sided causes are managed with a right hemicolectomy (with ileostomy and mucus fistula in some cases). Left-sided lesions are managed either by a two-stage approach consisting of resection and an end stoma (Hartmann's procedure) or a single-stage procedure involving resection and on table lavage with anastomosis. This has the advantage of a shorter hospital stay and avoidance of stoma.

Discussion

The most concerning sequelae of intestinal obstruction are the possibilities of visceral perforation or infarction. While small bowel obstruction may be managed conservatively, at least initially, large bowel obstruction carries a higher risk of perforation, and will generally need more aggressive management. Patients should be assessed regularly for clinical deterioration and bloods monitored for dehydration and electrolyte disturbances.

Key Points

1. Multiple etiologies lead to this patient presentation. Distinction between large and small bowel obstruction can often be made by history and examination with radiographs.
2. Complete a full examination noting previous surgery; do not neglect the hernia orifices and a rectal examination.
3. Obstruction can lead to significant fluid shift, and resuscitation must be tailored accordingly with regular monitoring of electrolytes.
4. Patients must be regularly assessed for signs of perforation or ischemia and surgery planned immediately.
5. Always consent patients for bowel resection and stoma formation.

Clinical Case Scenario 4: Lower GI Bleeding

Case Presentation

A 75 year old man presents to the accident and emergency department with severe rectal bleeding. He has passed close to a liter of blood in the last 4 h which he describes as mostly fresh looking and not mixed with the stools. He complains of some lower abdominal discomfort and denies any change in his bowel habit. He has a history of cardiac disease and is currently taking an aspirin tablet daily. On examination, he is distressed, tachypneic and apyrexial with a pulse of 120 bpm and a blood pressure of 100/80 mmHg.

Key Features of History and Examination

Lower gastrointestinal bleeding makes up approximately one-quarter of all gastrointestinal bleeding, ranging from minimal hematochezia (passage of bright red or maroon blood per rectum), melena (passage of black tarry stools per rectum, suggesting an upper gastrointestinal cause), to significant shock. There is a mortality of between 10% and 20% reported due to the significant comorbidities and hemodynamic instability in certain patients. Lower GI bleeding is defined as originating beyond the ligament of Trietz; however, an upper gastrointestinal cause must always be considered in brisk hematochezia (up to 11%).

The first priority in assessment is to look for any signs of hemodynamic instability and commence immediate resuscitation. The initial history should focus on identifying any specific risk factors, such as anticoagulant or NSAID use, and establishing the duration and frequency of the symptoms, the color of the stool (blood mixed with stool?), and any associated symptoms (fever, abdominal pain, vomiting). Other important aspects of the history include: previous episodes of bleeding and investigations performed, recent colonoscopy + polypectomy, symptoms suggestive of colorectal cancer (change in bowel habit, weight loss), inflammatory bowel disease, peptic ulcer disease, history of vascular disease/surgery, liver cirrhosis, family history of colonic pathology, and previous pelvic radiotherapy.

Examination must be thorough commencing at the oro/nasopharynx to exclude other sources of hemorrhage and including assessment for signs of chronic liver disease. Abdominal examination may identify a specific area of tenderness aiding the diagnosis. A careful digital rectal examination must be performed to exclude any obvious anorectal cause (hemorrhoids) and confirm the color of the blood/stool.

TABLE 1.4 Differential diagnosis of hamateochezia

Description	Incidence (%)	Possible causes
Upper gastrointestinal bleeding	0–11	Peptic ulcer disease
Small bowel bleeding	2–9	Meckel's diverticulum
		Mesenteric infarction
		Aortoenteric fistula
Anorectal cause	4–10	Anal fissure
		Hemorrhoids
		Solitary rectal ulcer
Neoplasia	11–14	Polyps
		Carcinoma
Colitis	2–30	Ischemic
		Infective
		Radiation
		Inflammatory bowel disease
Vascular	9–21	Angiodysplasia
Other	17–40	Diverticulosis

The differential diagnosis of hematochezia is listed in Table 1.4.

Principles of Acute Management

Management of lower gastrointestinal bleeding is based on the following principles:

Initial Assessment and Resuscitation

Patients require high flow oxygen, two wide bore intravenous cannulas, and fluid administration according to assessment of hemodynamic status. Patients with compromise should have a urinary catheter placed for fluid status monitoring. Certain high-risk patients may require transfer to the critical care department for invasive monitoring. Immediate investigations performed include the following:

Blood Tests

Initial blood tests include FBC (anemia, raised WCC, platelet count), clotting screen, group and save/cross match, U&Es (uremia – disproportionate to creatinine rise in upper GI causes due to digestion of blood proteins), and LFTs (chronic liver disease).

Locating the Bleeding Source and Therapeutic Intervention to Stop Bleeding

Oesophagogastroduodenoscopy (OGD)

In patients with significant hematochezia and hemodynamic instability, an OGD should be performed first to exclude an upper GI cause.

Sigmoidoscopy/Colonoscopy

A rigid sigmoidoscopy can be performed on all patients at admission to exclude obvious anorectal causes. A colonoscopy is the preferred choice of investigation with a diagnostic yield in acute bleeding of 89–97% of cases. It has the advantage of therapeutic interventions such as injection therapy, laser photocoagulation, and metallic clip application.

Nuclear Scintigraphy

This technetium-based scan is a sensitive method for detecting gastrointestinal bleeding at a rate of 0.1–0.5 mL/min. Images can be obtained for up to 24 h making a useful investigation in cases of intermittent bleeding.

Mesenteric Angiography

This technique can detect active bleeding when the rate is at least 0.5–1.0 mL/min. The specificity is 100% with a sensitivity of 48%. Therapeutic options include infusion of vasopressin and embolization. A complication rate of 9% is reported.

Surgery

The main indications for surgery include cases where bleeding is related to neoplasia, where the source is identified and conservative measures failed, in significant bleeding where the source has not been identified. Blind segmental colectomy is associated with a high morbidity and mortality; if the bleeding site is not localized, a subtotal colectomy should be performed.

Discussion

Lower gastrointestinal bleeding is less common than upper gastrointestinal bleeding, but with increasing age and comorbidities is associated with significant morbidity and mortality. Acute bleeding stops spontaneously in 80–85% of cases with a source not identified in 10–20%.

Five Key Points

1. The severity of lower gastrointestinal bleeding can be variable. High-risk patients of advanced age with multiple comorbidities should be identified early
2. Bleeding will stop spontaneously in 80–85% of cases.
3. Initial assessment and urgent resuscitation is the priority.
4. An OGD should be performed early to exclude an upper gastrointestinal cause.
5. Colonoscopy is the preferred diagnostic and therapeutic technique with angiography useful in cases of hemodynamic instability.

Clinical Case Scenario 5: Acute Pancreatitis

Case Presentation

A 50-year-old man presents to the accident and emergency department in the middle of the night with severe constant epigastric pain radiating to the back, associated with vomiting and anorexia. He has had one episode of diarrhea and no urinary symptoms. On examination, he is pyrexial at 38.2°C with a pulse of 111 bpm. Examination reveals severe tenderness of the central abdomen with guarding.

Key Features of History and Examination

Differential diagnosis of acute pancreatitis:

- Acute cholecystitis
- Acute cholangitis
- Peptic ulcer disease (perforation)
- Myocardial infarction
- Pneumonia
- Chronic pancreatitis

Gallstones and alcohol make up over 80% of the causes of acute pancreatitis. Other causes include drugs 2% (steroids, thiazide diuretics), trauma (post ERCP – 4%), metabolic (hyperlipidemia, hypercalcemia) autoimmune, viral infection (HIV/mumps) and structural (pancreatic divisum). All effort should be made within the history to identify the etiological factor. A majority of patients suffer a mild attack resolving within a few days. However, up to 20% of cases can have a significant systemic inflammatory response affecting cardiac, respiratory, and renal systems. For this reason, it is essential to fully assess comorbidities of the patients as they will likely affect the outcome.

On examination, patients are often in obvious pain. The presence of shock with a tachycardia, tachypnea, and cold peripheries is not uncommon. Abdominal examination reveals upper abdominal tenderness and guarding. Jaundice can be found (common bile duct stones) in about one-quarter of cases. Bruising may be seen in the periumbilical region (Cullen's sign) or flank (Grey Turner's sign) indicative of severe hemorrhagic pancreatitis with tracking of exudate. Repeated assessment of these patients is essential in prognosing the course of the disease and identifying any complications early.

Principles of Acute Management

Investigations are performed for both diagnosis and stratification of severity.

Blood Tests

The diagnosis is confirmed by detecting an elevated serum amylase or lipase. Serum amylase testing is widespread, although it is not specific for pancreatitis. A value of >1,000 u or four times the upper limit of normal is regarded as diagnostic. Other conditions such as perforated viscus or ischemic bowel can also give a rise in the amylase. Serum lipase is a more sensitive test for diagnosing pancreatitis with a longer serum half-life although less widespread. Urea and electrolytes should be checked for signs of renal impairment. LFTs can be abnormal in gallstone pancreatitis (ALT, ALP, and bilirubin). Clotting profile should be checked in cases of jaundice. CRP is also a useful predictor of severe pancreatitis (>150 mg/L at 48 h).

Erect CXR/AXR

To exclude perforated viscus

US Abdomen

Useful initial test in identifying etiology (gallstones)

CT Scan

This test is always indicated in patients with acute severe pancreatitis to assess for fluid collections and necrosis.

Severity stratification should be performed within 48 h of admission (see Table 1.5). A score of 3 or more usually predicts severe pancreatitis.

The management of mild pancreatitis is supportive consisting of intravenous fluids, catheterisation, analgesia (can require PCA),

TABLE 1.5 Scoring systems for acute pancreatitis

Glasgow criteria	Ranson criteria
Age > 55 years	Age > 55 years
WCC > 15 × 10⁹/L	WCC > 16 × 10⁹/L
Blood glucose > 10 nmol/L	Blood glucose > 11.1 nmol/L
Lactate dehydrogenase > 600 IU/L	Lactate dehydrogenase > 350 IU/L
Aspartate transaminase > 200 IU/L	Aspartate transaminase > 250 IU/L
Albumin < 32 g/L	Calcium < 2 mmol/L[a]
Calcium < 2 mmol/L	Urea > 1.8 mmol/L rise[a]
Urea > 16 mmol/L	Base deficit > 4 mmol/L[a]
	Arterial pO_2 < 60 mmHg[a]

[a]During initial 48 h

high flow oxygen, nasogastric aspiration, and venous thromboembolism prophylaxis. Strict control of fluid balance and regular monitoring of cardiorespiratory status and electrolytes is necessary. Early enteral feeding is ideal preserving mucosal protection and preventing translocation of bacteria.

Patients with severe pancreatitis should be monitored on high dependency or intensive care units. Invasive monitoring is often required due to significant fluid shifts and to prevent multiorgan failure (MODS). Many patients require ventilatory support, inotropes, and short-term dialysis. In such cases, parenteral nutrition is often indicated. There is no proven role in the use of routine antibiotics, with overuse associated with superinfection with *Candida* species. A proven benefit is reported in cases of infected necrosis limiting duration to 14 days.

ERCP and sphincterotomy should be performed in the presence of cholangitis, with early ERCP improving the outcome of a majority of patients with severe gallstone pancreatitis. Acute fluid collections are immature collections of enzyme-rich fluid which rarely cause symptoms and usually do not require any specific treatment. Pseudocysts are walled-off mature collections persisting for >4 weeks. Cysts of >7 cm commonly cause symptoms such as pain or compression indicating intervention. Management options include percutaneous aspiration or endoscopic drainage. Surgery for larger pseudocysts involves either a cystogastrostomy or cystojejunostomy which can be performed laparoscopically.

Surgery for necrotizing pancreatitis should be reserved for infected necrosis due to the high mortality. Necrosectomy includes blunt debridement of necrotic tissue with the retroperitoneum. Approaches can be open, laparoscopic, or even percutaneously through a nephroscope.

Discussion

In 2005, the UK Working Party released guidelines on the management of acute pancreatitis [3]. Recommendations include the following:

- The etiology of acute pancreatitis should be determined in at least 80% of cases, and no more than 20% should be classified as idiopathic.
- All patients with severe acute pancreatitis should be managed in a high dependency unit or intensive therapy unit with full monitoring and systems support.
- Urgent therapeutic ERCP should be performed in patients with acute pancreatitis of suspected or proven gallstone etiology who satisfy the criteria for predicted or actual severe pancreatitis, or when there is cholangitis, jaundice, or a dilated common bile duct. The procedure is best carried out within the first 72 h after the onset of pain.
- All patients with biliary pancreatitis should undergo definitive management of gallstones during the same hospital admission, unless a clear plan has been made for definitive treatment within the next 2 weeks.
- All patients with persistent symptoms and greater than 30% pancreatic necrosis, and those with smaller areas of necrosis and clinical suspicion of sepsis, should undergo image-guided FNA to obtain material for culture 7–14 days after the onset of the pancreatitis.

Five Key Points

1. Gallstones and alcohol account for over 80% of the causes of acute pancreatitis.
2. Severity stratification must be performed within 48 h of admission.
3. Close monitoring of fluid balance and cardiorespiratory status is essential to identify complications early.
4. Antibiotic use should be reserved for cases of infected necrosis and limited to 14 days.
5. Definitive treatment for gallstones in cases of biliary pancreatitis should be performed within 2 weeks of admission.

References

1. Martin DJ, Vernon D, Toouli J. Surgical versus endoscopic treatment of bile duct stones. Cochrane Database Syst Rev. 2006;(2):CD003327. doi: 10.1002/14651858.CD003327.pub2.
2. Sauerland S, Lefering R, Neugebauer EAM. Laparoscopic versus open surgery for suspected appendicitis. Cochrane Database Syst Rev. 2004;(4):CD001546. doi: 10.1002/14651858.CD001546.pub2.
3. UK Working Party on Acute Pancreatitis. UK guidelines for the management of acute pancreatitis. Gut. 2005;54:1–9.

Chapter 2
Vascular Emergencies

Susan L. Drinkwater, Vikas A. Pandey, and Alun H. Davies

Introduction

Vascular surgery is a relatively new specialty that used to be encompassed by general surgery involves multidisciplinary diagnosis and surgical treatment of cardiovascular disease. Medical management, minimally invasive treatment, and open surgical cases are key components of this specialty.

Now a days, separate on call rosters usually exist for vascular surgeons, as opposed to 10 years ago, when the general surgeon managed all vascular emergencies. Despite this, most junior trainees will often be the first point of contact, while on call.

S.L. Drinkwater (✉)
Department of Vascular Surgery,
Royal Preston Hospital, Lancashire, UK
e-mail: susan.drinkwater@lthtr.nhs.uk

V.A. Pandey, M.D., FRCS
Regional Vascular Unit, St. Mary's Hospital,
Imperial College Healthcare NHS Trust, London, UK

A.H. Davies, M.A., DM, FRCS, FHEA, FEBVS, FACPh
Department of Vascular Surgery, Charing Cross Hospital,
Imperial College Healthcare NHS Trust, London, UK

Faculty of Medicine, Charing Cross Hospital,
Imperial College School of Medicine, London, UK

I. Shergill et al. (eds.), *Surgical Emergencies in Clinical Practice*, 25
DOI 10.1007/978-1-4471-2876-2_2,
© Springer-Verlag London 2013

Because of the vital importance of time – ischemia from vascular injury may potentially result in loss of limb, loss of function, or loss of life – all junior trainees will be expected to have an excellent working knowledge of vascular conditions, as well as having a good understanding of expeditious management of vascular emergencies.

In this chapter, potentially life- and limb-threatening clinical cases are presented, with an emphasis on urgent recognition, through key features in the history and examination. The principles of acute management of these conditions are presented to avoid loss of limb, and loss of life, in day-to-day clinical practice.

Clinical Case Scenario 1: Ruptured Aortic Aneurysm (AAA)

Case Presentation

A 72-year-old hypertensive man presents with a 12-h history of severe and acute abdominal pain, radiating to the left flank, followed by collapse. On arrival in the emergency department, he appears pale, sweaty, and is tachycardic but normotensive. His pain persists. He is thought to have renal colic and is sent for a CT kidneys, ureters, and bladder (KUB) which shows a ruptured aortic aneurysm.

Key Features of History and Examination

Abdominal aortic aneurysm is most common in elderly male patients, but it does also occur in older women and may occur in younger patients where there is a genetic component. Smoking, hypertension, and hypercholesterolemia are all risk factors, as is a family history of the condition, so remember to ask about this or a family history of sudden death. Patients may have reported an abdominal pulsation. Often, there is a period of collapse, after which they regain consciousness and are hemodynamically stable. This is a result of a "herald bleed" contained within the retroperitoneal space and is associated with pain which is usually, but not always, in the left flank. It can be confused with renal colic. The patient may be too unwell or unconscious and not able to provide much by way of history. The possibility of ruptured abdominal aortic aneurysm must be considered in all patients even if the aneurysm is not palpable. The aorta is a deeply placed organ, and even a large aneurysm may not be palpable through a well-padded abdominal wall. Beware of a ruptured iliac aneurysm and/or thoracic aneurysm. There may be other clues on examination, such as prominent popliteal artery pulsations. Any patient with a known aortic aneurysm presenting with abdominal pain, back pain, or collapse should be assumed to have ruptured until proven otherwise. An aortic aneurysm may be symptomatic but may not have ruptured. Such patients are generally not discharged from hospital until their aortic aneurysm is repaired. Consider this in cases where the aortic aneurysm is tender, causing distal embolization or associated with an aorto-enteric fistula (rectal bleed, hematemesis).

Principles of Acute Management

If suspected, then all members of the surgical and anesthetic teams should be notified as soon as possible. Inform theaters so they can prepare theater personnel and necessary instruments. Call intensive care as the patient will most likely be transferred there postoperatively. The patient should be given high flow oxygen. Intravenous access (2×14 gauge venflons) should be obtained, a urinary catheter inserted, and blood collected for full blood count, urea and electrolytes, a coagulation profile (if clinically indicated), and blood for cross match. Many hematology departments have "ruptured aneurysm" or "massive bleed" protocols so activate these.

Resuscitate the patient carefully. A policy of "permissive hypotension" is usually adopted. This does not prohibit the use of fluids, but they should be given to maintain a systolic blood pressure of just above 80 mmHg. Blood is ideal.

Ensure adequate analgesia. Call the family and discuss with the patient if there is time and the patient is conscious.

Computerised tomography (CT) angiography will confirm the diagnosis, show the extent of the aneurysm, and allow for procedural planning. If there is local expertise available, the aneurysm is anatomically suitable, and the patient is sufficiently stable, they may benefit from an endovascular aneurysm repair.

It is very important to image the thoracic aorta as well in order to exclude thoracic aneurysm or dissection. Ultrasound is of limited use as it will confirm the presence of an abdominal aortic aneurysm but not whether it has ruptured. If unstable, the patient should be taken straight to theater. Similarly, if a patient is being transferred from a referring hospital with a proven ruptured aneurysm, there is no place for assessment or resuscitation in the emergency room of the receiving hospital, and any assessment should take place in the anesthetic room.

Discussion

The prevalence of abdominal aortic aneurysm increases with age and occurs in 7–8% of males over the age of 65. It is six times more common in men than in women, and this is why only men are invited to participate in screening in the United Kingdom. Rupture of an AAA is the seventh most common cause for male death in the United Kingdom. Preventing rupture by population screening will hopefully reduce this number as the outcomes for elective repair are much better than for emergency repair (mortality rates of 5% versus 50%, respectively). Sharing common risk factors, patients with aneurysmal disease may also have Coexisting occlusive disease, so a complete peripheral arterial assessment is required in these patients. This is of considerable importance as one of the risks of aortic surgery is limb ischemia. Coexisting popliteal or femoral aneurysms must be looked for on examination.

Currently, trials are underway comparing open versus endovascular repair of ruptured abdominal aortic aneurysms. Successful outcomes are reported following endovascular repair, but the patient may develop abdominal compartment syndrome and require a laparostomy. This strategy depends on local expertise. There is an overall mortality rate of 50% following open repair, and this has not changed over the last 50 years despite advances in anesthesia or intensive care. If stable, there is some evidence that outcomes are better if the patient is transferred to a unit with a vascular surgeon rather than attempting a repair by a nonvascular specialist.

The outcome following AAA repair is poor in the very elderly and in those patients who have suffered a concurrent cardiac arrest. It is also unfavorable in those patients persistently unconscious following initial circulatory collapse, and in these situations, a decision not to repair may be appropriate but can only be made by a senior vascular surgeon.

Clinical Case Scenario 2: Aortic Dissection

Case Presentation

A 50-year-old man presents with a sudden history of tearing chest pain, occurring centrally and radiating to his back. He describes this as the "worst pain" he has ever had. He is on treatment for hypertension, and his blood pressure on arrival was 230/110 mmHg. On arrival to the emergency department, he complains that his feet are cold and numb, he has ischemic legs, and is anuric.

Key Features of History and Examination

One of the main points in the history is the abrupt onset of pain that patients consistently describe as tearing in nature and frequently state is the worst they have ever experienced. They may be breathless or feel faint or give a history of collapse. The patient may give a history of hypertension and is usually hypertensive on arrival, as this is the commonest etiology. The patient may have marfanoid features (tall, high arched palate, arm span greater than height, arachnodactyly), or they may have a formal diagnosis of bicuspid aortic valve,

Turner's syndrome, Marfan's syndrome, Ehlers-Danlos syndrome, or another connective tissue disorder. Ask about a history of syphilis and cocaine use.

A full peripheral arterial examination should be performed, as the absence of distal pulses is a poor prognostic factor that indicates extensive disease. There may be a difference in the recorded blood pressure between the right and left arms and a slow radial pulse. The patient may present with neurological symptoms (paraplegia) or stroke. There may be abdominal pain or tenderness (visceral ischemia) or flank tenderness (renal ischemia), and there may be oliguria or anuria. An electrocardiogram (ECG) will be done to exclude a coronary event and is usually normal.

Principles of Acute Management

The first step is to suspect the diagnosis. Analgesia is essential, as is the swift pharmacological control of blood pressure which often requires consultation with a cardiologist. Management of aortic dissection is dependent on the classification, and although many classification systems exist, the Stanford classification is by far the easiest to remember. Dissections proximal to the left subclavian artery are termed Stanford type A and distal to the left subclavian, Stanford type B.

Type A aortic dissection requires *URGENT* cardiothoracic referral as the mortality rate from an untreated type A dissection is 1%/h (from acute aortic regurgitation and/or rupture, pericardial tamponade, and coronary ischemia). Type B dissection can be further classified into uncomplicated or complicated (associated with limb, visceral, spinal, or renal ischemia).

High flow oxygen should be administered, and intravenous access established with large bore cannulas. ECG should be performed and blood tests, including full blood count, urea and electrolytes, coagulation screen, and cross match. Liver function tests and amylase may provide clues to mesenteric perfusion, and an arterial blood gas is helpful. Creatine kinase (CK) is often helpful in complicated type B cases.

Tight blood pressure control is required. Intravenous beta-blockers are usually the first line of choice. Glyceryl trinitrate (GTN) infusions may be used but can cause headache if used for a prolonged period. Analgesia is also required, in the form of a patient-controlled analgesia (PCA).

Computerised tomographic angiography (CTA) should be performed urgently, and then a management plan worked out accordingly. Type A dissections require urgent aortic root replacement by a cardiothoracic surgeon. The majority of type B dissections can be managed conservatively, with tight blood pressure control and analgesia.

Complicated type B dissections, however, will require intervention. If the patient presents with single limb ischemia, then femoro-femoral cross-over bypass grafting may be indicated. If there is renal or mesenteric ischaemia paralysis, or even an aortic rupture, then the treatment of choice is endovascular stent grafting. Sometimes, a short covered stent can be placed over the intimal tear to close it and fenestrations created more distally to restore flow to the true lumen.

Discussion

Aortic dissection can occur in hypertensives and in patients with a family history. It is associated with Marfan's disease and bicuspid aortic valves. Sometimes, there are no predisposing factors known. There may be limb, gut, or renal ischemia depending on the extension of the dissection flap, all of which are poor prognostic factors.

This patient's prognosis is very poor, but fortunately many patients do very well with simple conservative measures for type B dissection. For most patients, the pain settles over a few days. If pain persists, they are thought to be at risk of rupture and endovascular intervention is indicated. Imaging is repeated usually after a fortnight to determine whether there has been expansion of the false lumen, which would be another indication to intervene. After 2 weeks, the dissection is termed "chronic." About 30% of patients with chronic dissection undergo aneurysmal change and so serial CTs are recommended (usually on an annual basis). The aorta remodels more effectively in the acute period rather than once the dissection is well established, and as there is no certain means of predicting which patients will develop late expansion, there are trials underway to determine whether all patients might benefit from endovascular stent grafting in the acute period.

Clinical Case Scenario 3: Acutely Ischaemic Limb

Case Presentation

A 53-year-old man comes into the accident and emergency department with a cold, white, numb foot. This came on very suddenly a couple of hours ago. He has never experienced any problems in the leg before. He is a smoker and hypertensive and suffers from the odd episode of palpitations but is otherwise well.

Key Features of History and Examination

A patient with an acutely ischemic limb will report symptoms that have typically come on within hours but less than 2 weeks (which would make it a critically ischemic limb). They may have risk factors for atherosclerosis (smoking, hypertension, diabetes, male gender, family history, hypercholesterolemia). They may have an arrhythmia and may or may not be anticoagulated with warfarin. Think about the silent MI as a source of embolus, particularly in a diabetic. They may have a history of previous vascular surgery and have a bypass graft or stent graft that has acutely occluded.

The presence or absence of pulses on the other side is a useful clue for determining etiology. Presence of pulses might indicate an embolus, absent pulses might indicate preexisting arterial disease, and a very prominent popliteal pulse might point the finger at an aneurysm. Check for an aortic aneurysm as an embolic source.

Classically, the patient presents with a limb that is painful, and perishingly cold, and may have parasthesia and paralysis. It is pale and pulseless on examination. Parasthesia and paralysis are signs that the leg is imminently threatened and may not be viable more than 6 h after onset of symptoms in the case of an acute embolism in a leg with previously normal vasculature. If there is preexisting peripheral vascular disease, collaterals may have developed, which means that the leg may remain viable for longer. The foot may not be pale, but may be mottled or dusky. The capillary refill time is of useful significance in a dusky leg. If delayed (if it takes longer to refill than it does to say "capillary refill"), this would indicate ischemia. Calf or anterior compartment tenderness is also a disturbing sign and would indicate muscle under threat. Fixed mottling (that does not blanch with pressure) and paralysis usually mean an unsalvageable limb.

Principles of Acute Management

The important points here are to accurately identify a limb at need of urgent intervention. There may only be a small time frame when the limb might be salvageable. The patient may have had a recent coronary event, and if the event was embolic, be at risk of further embolization (stroke, mesenteric ischemia).

The patient will need rapid assessment and appropriate referral. Analgesia is important, and the patient will usually require intravenous opiates. Bloods should be sent for full blood count, urea and electrolytes (prior to intravenous contrast), coagulation screen (baseline), group and save, and troponin (if recent onset chest pain or they are diabetic). ECG should be performed to determine whether the patient is in sinus rhythm and to exclude a myocardial infarction. If in atrial fibrillation, they will need rate controlling.

Anticoagulate with intravenous heparin as the patient may have had an embolus, and they may need urgent arteriography or surgery. Give a 5,000 unit bolus intravenously and then start an infusion. If available, an urgent CT angiogram or arterial duplex by a skilled vascular technician is invaluable and may be all the imaging that is required prior to surgery.

If no imaging is available, the limb is white, and the patient appears to have had a very acute embolic event, it may be appropriate to take the patient straight to the operating theater at this point, without additional imaging, and perform an angiogram "on-table" if necessary. A femoral embolectomy may be performed easily in an unwell patient under local anesthetic.

If there is diagnostic uncertainty and there are no runoff vessels on the duplex scan, and there is thought that thrombolysis might be indicated, or that the patient might benefit from radiological intervention, an arteriogram may be performed.

Discussion

An acutely ischemic limb may be a result of trauma, embolus, in situ arterial thrombosis, or a thrombosed popliteal aneurysm. It can often be very difficult to identify an acutely ischemic limb. The key is to identify the limb at risk from the limb that is unsalvageable, as trying to reperfuse a nonviable limb is extremely hazardous for the patient. Prompt decisions are necessary. The patient may be very unwell following a recent coronary event. Always consider whether fasciotomies may be necessary.

The majority of embolic events come from a cardiac source and an echocardiogram should be performed, although this may be normal. It may be necessary to image the aorta with CT to look for an alternative source of embolization (aneurysm, ulcer, atheroma).

If the patient presents with a popliteal aneurysm, they will need to be screened for abdominal aortic aneurysm and the popliteal on the other side as these frequently coexist.

Clinical Case Scenario 4: Transient Ischemic Attack

Case Presentation

A 65-year-old man is brought in by his family after developing weakness of his right arm and slurring of his speech. He describes a similar episode 2 weeks previously that resolved over an hour. On further questioning, he describes transient visual loss that affected his left eye. These symptoms improve over the course of the day.

Key Features of History and Examination

Emboli originating from the internal carotid artery cause ischemic changes in the territory of the middle cerebral artery or ophthalmic artery. These manifest as symptoms including contralateral limb weakness or sensory disturbance. Ipsilateral monocular blindness (amaurosis fugax, typically described as a "curtain obstructing vision in one eye") is a result of emboli in the ophthalmic artery and is usually transient. Slurring of the speech may be present with left hemispheric TIA or stroke (95% of right-handed and 70% of left-handed people have their speech center located in the left cerebral hemisphere). A transient ischemic attack by definition fully resolves within 24 h. The patient will have one or more for atherosclerosis risk factors. On neurological examination, there may be weakness of the upper or lower limbs or both. The patient may be hyperreflexic with an upgoing plantar response on the affected side. Sensory inattention may be present together with dysarthria or dysphasia. A carotid bruit is sometimes, but not always, present, and its presence or absence is not helpful (it may be absent with a severe stenosis of the internal carotid artery or may be present and associated with a mild stenosis or actually be emanating from the external carotid artery). There may be stigmata of related cardiovascular disease (i.e., sternotomy incision from previous CABG, absent foot pulses, aneurysmal disease).

Principles of Acute Management

Although often referred to the internal medical team, surgeons should be adept at the investigation and management of patients with transient ischemic attacks. Prompt management of transient ischemic attacks can prevent stroke in approximately 43% of patients within 7 days of the index event. All patients should have bloods including glucose and inflammatory markers (the latter may point to an arteritic process), and ECG should be performed to exclude cardiac ischemia or arrhythmia or occult cardiac pathology. A CT scan of the brain may be performed if there is clinical suspicion of a hemorrhagic stroke (accounting for 20% of all strokes). Antiplatelet therapy should be commenced in all patients unless contraindicated.

Duplex ultrasonography is the investigation of choice in assessment of carotid disease. It is a low cost, noninvasive investigation; however, it is not readily available out of hours. In such cases, CT or magnetic resonance angiography of the carotid arteries may be performed. There is good evidence that CEA (combined with medical therapy) is superior to best medical therapy when the degree of ICA stenosis is greater than 70%. Surgery should be scheduled on the next available elective operating list and certainly within 7 days of the index TIA in uncomplicated cases. If the patient is not receiving clopidogrel, they should receive a 75 mg stat dose the evening before surgery, as this has been shown to reduce the incidence of perioperative embolization. Patients with subthreshold stenosis (<70%) should be managed with best medical therapy. Any cases that are not clear cut should be discussed at a multidisciplinary team meeting, as should all operative cases if logistically practical.

Patients admitted with a stroke in evolution, progressive hemiplegia, or crescendo TIAs should be considered for emergency CEA. Patients admitted with these conditions should be anticoagulated with unfractionated heparin prior to surgery. Patients thrombolyzed for stroke as a result of thrombotic occlusion of the ICA may have an underlying stenosis unmasked by thrombolysis. Such patients should also be treated in the same manner and have an early CEA.

Discussion

In this modern era, it is not unusual for specialist vascular surgical teams to be involved in the management of transient ischemic attack. CEA is no longer a "cold" elective case, and health services worldwide are employing a more aggressive approach to its management. Increasingly CEA is being performed out of hours and at weekends. The modern surgeon working in a vascular unit should be adept at performing neurological examination, and the threshold for operating should be lowered if there is any suggestion of ongoing neurological deterioration. In cases of TIA related to atherosclerotic disease, the benefits of CEA are greatest in the first 24 h. Patients should be given antiplatelet medication (aspirin, dipyridamole, clopidogrel) if they are not already receiving this, and some patients will require intravenous unfractionated heparin prior to expedited surgery.

Clinical Case Scenario 5: Extensive or Proximal DVT

Case Presentation

A 35-year-old pianist presents with a history of a swollen, purple right arm a day after doing some DIY. He gives no significant past medical history.

Key Features of History and Examination

Deep venous thrombosis is common and about 50% will have no symptoms or signs. Proximal or very extensive deep venous thromboses, may benefit from intervention to prevent post-thrombotic syndrome. The patient may give no significant history, but may, with upper limb deep venous thrombosis, report heavy lifting or repetitive activity (such as rowing, painting, horse riding) in the preceding days (Paget-Schroetter syndrome), and they may be particularly muscular. They may give a family history of thrombophilia, or report previous deep vein thromboses or recurrent miscarriages. A careful history must also include other risk factors for deep venous thrombosis (obesity, travel, injury, immobility, oral contraceptive pill, smoking), and the possibility of an underlying malignancy must be considered. The thrombosis of course may be secondary to central venous catheterization. The patient may present with a swollen arm or leg. The swelling will generally affect the whole limb. This may be associated with pain, but it may not be particularly painful. There are signs of venous congestion, with blue or purple discolouration, and increased capillary refill time. The limb may feel cool from the edema, which may make pulses difficult to palpate, and the discoloration may fool the unwary into thinking this might be an ischemic limb. The rapid capillary refill is the clue here. The classic description of phlegmasia cerula dolens is of a swollen discolored limb, but the presentation may be more subtle. In very severe cases, there may be associated arterial spasm (phlegmasia alba dolens) and the limb does appear ischemic. There may be dilated superficial veins.

Principles of Acute Management

The first step is to prevent thrombus propagation or pulmonary embolization, and so the patients needs to be anticoagulated. This is usually with a therapeutic dose of low-molecular-weight heparin, but intravenous heparin may be appropriate if the patient is being considered for thrombolysis. A venous duplex scan is the most sensitive and specific test, but a CT scan with venous phase contrast may be used if duplex is unavailable. Bloods should be sent for D dimers and clotting screen, to screen for an underlying malignancy (FBC, U&E, LFTs, bone profile, CRP, tumor markers) and a thrombophilia screen (protein C, protein S, antithrombin III, activated protein C resistance), prior to commencing anticoagulation.

The limb should be elevated and compression applied, whether this be a full length compression stocking or a intermittent pneumatic compression device.

A decision is then made as to whether the patient will benefit from thrombolysis. Proximal deep venous thromboses have a significant (25–40%) risk of developing into post-thrombotic syndrome. This can mean a permanently swollen limb, and in the case of the lower limb, skin changes and venous ulceration. These sequelae can take years to develop.

For this reason, older patients, who are more likely to have a stroke from thrombolysis, and are more likely to have an underlying malignancy, are not usually offered thrombolysis. Thrombolysis is more likely to be offered in the dominant arm, in a younger person, and with a hobby or occupation that requires precise movements (such as a musician). Recent surgery, active peptic ulceration, or other bleeding diatheses are contraindication for thrombolysis and must be determined in the history.

Thought needs to be given to whether there is an underlying anatomical cause for the thrombosis, such as thoracic outlet syndrome, and chest and cervical spine X-rays are recommended for upper limb thromboses, to look for a cervical rib. At a later stage, an MRI scan is recommended, but this is not part of the acute management.

Once thrombolysis has been successfully achieved, further imaging is required to identify and treat any underlying anatomical abnormality, be it a cervical rib or band or compression from the iliac artery (May-Thurner lesion).

Discussion

One may not think of deep venous thrombosis as a vascular emergency, as it is usually managed by physicians. Certainly, the most dangerous complication of DVT is pulmonary embolism. However, patients with axillary/subclavian venous thromboses or even extensive iliofemoral deep vein thromboses may suffer significant morbidity from post-thrombotic syndrome and may well benefit from emergency thrombolysis, which explains why they are included in this category.

The key thing to consider here is that about 25% of patients will be diagnosed with a malignancy within 12 months of presenting with an upper limb DVT. It is very important, therefore, to take a careful history and examination.

This particular patient, who is a professional musician, would benefit from thrombolysis, even if the symptoms were relatively minor.

Five Key Learning Points

1. Think of the diagnosis of a ruptured aortic aneurysm. Remember, not all presentations are typical. Resuscitate with blood.
2. Aortic dissection requires tight blood pressure control, analgesia, and rapid imaging, as urgent intervention may be required.
3. An acutely ischemic leg may be secondary to an embolism, an acute thrombosis, or a thrombosed aneurysm.
4. Crescendo TIAs should be considered a surgical emergency.
5. Consider whether a patient with proximal DVT may benefit from thrombolysis.

Chapter 3
Endocrine Emergencies

Tahwinder Upile, Navdeep Upile, and Jaspal Mahil

Introduction

Endocrine surgery is commonly carried out in many hospitals, including thyroidectomy, parathyroidectomy, and adrenal surgery. Although we have selected specifically difficult endocrine management problems, it must be remembered that basic surgical management must be adhered to when dealing with the complications of endocrine surgery. For instance, after thyroid or parathyroid surgery, an increasing neck swelling will indicate

T. Upile, B.Sc. (hons), M.Sc., M.S., M.D., FRCS (Gen Surg), FRCS (OTO), FRCS (ORL-HNS), DFFP, FHEA, MRCGP (✉)
Department of ENT, Barnet and Chase Farm Hospital,
Enfield, Greater London, UK

Head and Neck Unit, University College London Hospitals,
Greater London, UK
e-mail: mrtupile@yahoo.com

N. Upile, BMedSci MRCS
Cancer Research Centre, University of Liverpool,
200 London Rd, L3 9TA, UK
e-mail: nupile@liverpool.ac.uk

J. Mahil, B.Sc. (hons), MRCGP, DFFP
Department of ENT, Barnet and Chase Farm Hospital,
Enfield, Greater London, UK
e-mail: mrtupile@yahoo.com

I. Shergill et al. (eds.), *Surgical Emergencies in Clinical Practice*,   41
DOI 10.1007/978-1-4471-2876-2_3,
© Springer-Verlag London 2013

an impending compartment syndrome due to perhaps hemorrhage. The consequence of this is potential airways compromise which can be easily treated by early removal of sutures and evacuation of hematoma, if necessary. Similarly, bilateral recurrent laryngeal nerve damage after surgery may result in bilateral vocal cord adduction and loss of airway in the perioperative phase which must be rapidly treated by either intubation or removal of sutures and tracheostomy. Furthermore, when dealing with potentially hormone-secreting tumors such as pheochromocytomas, care must be taken to exclude similar tumors in other locations. It is essential that multidisciplinary care is entered into early, and that when required, appropriate referral is made at the opportune time to more senior and/or specialist teams. The current national trend appears to be that much of the thyroid and parathyroid surgery is now carried out by ENT surgeons rather than general, endocrine, or other discipline head and neck surgeons. This is based upon the ability for thorough preoperative assessment (including voice measures and nerve function) and postoperative rehabilitation (speech and voice) and the treatment of possible complications that is now possible by otolaryngologists.

We have selected the cases based upon their frequency of presentation, need for correct initial management, and due to the medicolegal consequences of poor management. Other more complex surgical emergencies may be found in specialty-specific texts. Also note replacement of electrolytes must include appropriate monitoring, which can include cardiac monitoring. Furthermore, many trusts have generated specific protocols that should also be referred to.

Clinical Case Scenario 1: Hypercalcemia

Case Presentation

A 75-year-old man presents with confusion, incontinence, lethargy, weakness, constipation, abdominal pain, with nausea and vomiting 2 weeks after he had a transurethral resection of prostate (TURP). He has atrial fibrillation and has been on warfarin. Clinical examination revealed a nontender abdomen and hard nodular, malignant-feeling prostate. A biochemical profile revealed a plasma calcium of 3.375 mmol/L and raised ALP. Histology reports, brought to your attention by the ward sister, reveal a newly diagnosed prostate cancer at TURP. Two weeks after correction of his biochemical imbalance, a bone scan reveals multiple bone metastases from prostate cancer.

Key Points in History and Examination

Features of hypercalcemia may manifest themselves in different ways, remembered by the "moans, stones, and abdominal groans" trilogy.

General

Patients present with lethargy, weakness, anorexia, and bone pains.

Gastrointestinal Symptoms

Typically they present with constipation, nausea and vomiting, peptic ulceration, and abdominal pain.

Renal Symptoms

Polyuria and/or polydipsia are the commonest symptoms, but they may also present as acute renal failure, renal tubular damage with hypokalemia, dehydration, and sodium loss.

Psychological Symptoms

Common symptoms are depression and dementia.

Other Features

Occasionally, only abnormal calcification (urolithiasis, conjunctival flare, and chondrocalcinosis) and cardiac arrhythmias may be the presenting features.

PTH should normally be suppressed by a high serum calcium; however, possible biochemical indicators of hyperparathyroidism are normal or low albumin, a normal or reduced phosphate, a raised PTH (or inappropriately in the normal range), and a normal urea. A biochemical constellation of low plasma albumin, low chloride, raised phosphate, raised alkaline phosphatase, alkalosis, and hypokalemia may possibly indicate malignancy.

Principles of Acute Management

Immediate referral for multidisciplinary management, with medical input and/or intensive care support, should be given if clinically indicated. Acute management aims to intra-vascular circulating volume and renal calcium excretion, reducing bone resorption and targeting the underlying disease process. If the calcium is >3.5 mmol/L, the aim is to reduce the calcium.

Biochemical testing: Repeat U&Es, creatinine, calcium, magnesium, phosphate and alkaline phosphatase.

The initial treatment for the hypercalcemia is with intravenous normal saline (e.g., 0.9% NaCl, between 4 and 6 L/24 h) with the cautious addition of a loop diuretic (e.g., frusemide 40 mg/12 h) with monitoring of hemodynamic and electrolyte status. Any attendant hypokalemia and hypomagnesemia should be corrected to help alleviate symptoms and promote urinary calcium losses. At first, the serum calcium will fall rapidly; however, the effect lasts only as long as the infusion and diuresis continues. Correction of hypokalemia and hypomagnesemia using intravenous supplements with regular monitoring of plasma sodium, potassium, magnesium, urea, and CVP are required.

Further treatments are directed at reducing bone resorption due to enhanced osteoclastic bone resorption by using a bisphosphonate (e.g., pamidronate over the next few days with maximum effect at 1 week) or other agents. Additionally, glucocorticoids (e.g., prednisolone 40–60 mg/24 h) are effective in hypercalcemia associated with hematological malignancy (lymphoma, multiple myeloma) and in diseases such as sarcoidosis and vitamin D toxicity. Finally, hemodialysis against low-calcium dialysate is recommended for the dialysis-dependent hypercalcemic patient. Chemotheraphy may help reduce hypercalcemia of malignant origin.

Discussion

The underlying cause of the hypercalcemia must be identified and then treated, with general measures aimed at lowering the serum calcium by reducing the use of thiazide diuretics and immobilization (raises serum calcium). Generous rehydration and electrolyte replacement promotes calcium excretion and avoid extracellular volume depletion. The commonest reason for severe hypercalcemia is malignancy, usually metastatic to bones. This should be identified and appropriately treated. In this case, hormone therapy for metastatic prostate cancer was initiated with improvement of calcium levels over the following few weeks. The second commonest cause is due to a raised parathyroid hormone (PTH), and if this is the case, subsequent referral for urgent parathyroidectomy should be made.

Clinical Case Scenario 2: Diabetic Ketoacidosis

Case Presentation

A 47-year-old poorly compliant patient with insulin-dependent diabetes presents with right iliac fossa pain. He is appropriately diagnosed and treated for appendicitis. One day after surgery, he is found to have persistently raised BMs on the surgical ward, ranging from 17 to 25, and has been noted to becoming increasingly drowsy over the past few hours. Ketones are detected on urine dipsticks, and the nursing staff on the ward contact the on call surgical trainee for urgent advice, worried that he may have developed diabetic ketoacidosis (DKA).

Key Points in History and Examination

History

Look for symptoms of vomiting, abdominal pain, headache, thirst, and polyuria. He may have had similar episodes in the past, in view of poor compliance with insulin.

Examination

Assess respiratory rate, as he may have developed Kussmaul breathing. Check blood pressure for hypotension. His breath may have a characteristic "fruity smell" almost pathognomonic for DKA.

Investigations

Urgently check urine for signs of infection and send off MSU. Check full blood count for WCC, urgent U + Es, as well as serum glucose. If DKA is suspected, urgent ABG is indicated to look for low pH and low serum bicarbonate. CXR should be done to exclude chest infection as an underlying cause, and urgent ECG is indicated to look for high serum potassium – peaked T waves progressing to widened QRS progressing to VT.

Principles of Acute Management

The patient is very unwell and urgent multidisciplinary care is required with the help of physicians and intensive care doctors. Urgent resuscitation, in the form of intravenous fluids (normal saline) and intravenous antibiotics, should be commenced. A urinary catheter should be inserted for urine output monitoring. Insulin replacements should then be administered, initially via an intravenous infusion at a rate determined by the plasma glucose – sliding scale insulin with diabetic nurse specialist involvement. Subcutaneous insulin should not be given, due to variable absorption, in the emergency situation.

Discussion

Diabetic patients being admitted for emergency surgery require intravenous control of their blood glucose irrespective of the severity of their diabetes – protocols are likely to vary between hospitals. This case, similar to those cases seen on surgical wards, is imminently preventable using this approach. One should discontinue previous diabetic therapy. The administration of insulin by infusion pump (e.g., administered from a stock solution of 1 L of 10% dextrose 12 hourly with a 20 mmol potassium supplement) should be regulated according to the blood glucose level and should aim to keep the serum glucose concentrations between 5 and 10 mM. The blood glucose should be measured regularly on an hourly basis (and the insulin infusion rate altered accordingly). Intravenous glucose control should be continued until the patient is eating again. Thereafter, the normal diabetic regime may be recommenced.

Clinical Case Scenario 3: Pheochromocytoma Emergency

Case Presentation

A 35-year-old hypertensive man presents with the following symptoms at anesthetic induction: headache, visual disturbances, diaphoresis, palpitations, tremor, nausea, weakness, anxiety, epigastric pain, constipation, and weight loss. He has several pedunculated skin lesions (neurofibromas) and more than six café-au-lait spots and a scar on his neck. Further examination reveals pyrexia, hypertension, postural hypotension, tachycardia, pulmonary edema, cardiomyopathy, and ileus. Biochemical profiles reveal hyperglycemia.

Key Features of History and Examination

The biological effects of catecholamines are well known; however, pheochromocytomas may also produce calcitonin, opioid peptides, somatostatin, corticotropin (may cause Cushing's syndrome), and vasoactive intestinal peptide (may cause watery diarrhea). Stimulation of alpha-adrenergic receptors results in elevated blood pressure; increased cardiac contractility, glycogenolysis, gluconeogenesis; and intestinal relaxation. Stimulation of beta-adrenergic receptors results in an increase in heart rate and contractility.

In the history, various familial syndromes may be present.

MEN 2A Syndrome (Sipple's Syndrome)

Medullary thyroid carcinoma, hyperparathyroidism, pheochromocytomas, and Hirschsprung disease.

MEN 2B Syndrome

Medullary thyroid carcinoma, pheochromocytoma, mucosal neurofibromatosis, intestinal ganglioneuromatosis, Hirschsprung disease, and marfanoid body habitus.

Von Hippel Lindau (VHL) Disease

Pheochromocytoma, cerebellar hemangioblastoma, renal cell carcinoma, renal and pancreatic cysts, and epididymal cystadenomas. This syndrome is present in nearly 19% of patients with pheochromocytomas.

Neurofibromatosis

This is characterized by congenital anomalies (often benign tumors) of the skin, nervous system, bones, and endocrine glands. Only 1% of patients with neurofibromatosis have been found to have pheochromocytomas, but as many as 5% of patients with pheochromocytomas have been found to have neurofibromatosis. Other neuroectodermal disorders associated with pheochromocytomas include tuberous sclerosis (Bourneville's disease, epiloia) and Sturge-Weber syndrome.

Principles of Acute Management

High circulating catecholamine levels stimulate alpha-receptors on blood vessels and cause vasoconstriction. Alpha-adrenergic blockade, in particular, is required to control blood pressure and prevent a hypertensive crisis. Surgical resection of the tumor is the treatment of choice and usually results in cure of the hypertension. Prudent treatment with alpha- and beta-blockers is required. Medical therapy is used for preoperative preparation prior to surgery, acute hypertensive crises, and primary therapy for patients with metastatic pheochromocytomas. Preoperative preparation requires combined alpha- and beta-blockade to control blood pressure and to prevent an intraoperative hypertensive crisis.

General measures: The following measures can be undertaken preoperatively to control blood pressure and prevent intraoperative hypertensive crises. It is essential to liaise with the anesthetist who will be undertaking the case.

1. Start alpha-blockade, for example, phenoxybenzamine 7–10 days preoperatively to allow for expansion of blood volume.
2. The patient should undergo volume expansion with isotonic sodium chloride solution. Encourage liberal electrolyte replacement.
3. Initiate a beta-blocker only after adequate alpha-blockade. If beta-blockade is started prematurely, unopposed alpha-stimulation could precipitate a hypertensive crisis.
4. Administer the last doses of oral alpha- and beta-blockers on the morning of surgery.

Discussion

Pheochromocytoma, presenting as an emergency, in the absence of previous history is extremely rare. Most cases are known about and cause symptoms prior to adrenal surgery. If there is any doubt at time of induction of anesthesia, surgery should be abandoned, pending appropriate treatment and investigation of possible underlying disease.

Clinical Case Scenario 4: Hypocalcemia After Thyroid Surgery

Case Presentation

A 53-year-old female presents for a completion thyroidectomy and Level 6 neck dissection following a left thyroid lobectomy for papillary carcinoma found in a $3 \times 2 \times 2$ nodule. The original histology showed vascular and capsular invasion and the inclusion of the left glands in the specimen. During very difficult surgery on a previous and recently operated site, the parathyroids were not clearly identified. The recurrent laryngeal nerves were identified and preserved. The patient recovered from anesthesia but within a few hours complained of muscle cramps with carpopedal spasms and perioral tingling.

Key Features in History and Examination

A previous history of central neck surgery may suggest the diagnosis of hypocalcemia. Clinical examination reveals facial muscle excitability on percussion over the parotid area (Chvostek's sign) and ipsilateral capal spasm on blood pressure measurement (Trousseau sign). Repeat biochemical testing including liver function tests and serum phosphatase is advised.

Management

The patient's management will depend upon the severity of the hypocalcemia. Mild symptoms may require calcium supplement in the order of 5 mmol/6 h. While for severe symptoms, intravenous calcium gluconate (2.25 mmol), that is, 10 mL (10%) may be given over 30 min. Repeating the treatment may be required, depending upon symptoms and biochemistry. Bolus injections are reserved for life-threatening circumstances. Alfacalcidol at 0.5–1 ug/24 h orally may be useful.

Discussion

A similar situation may arise after laryngectomy/laryngo-pharngectomy/gastric transposition (stomach pull-up) surgery or any local surgery after radiotherapy since the vascular supply to the parathyroid glands may become compromised. Even when the parathyroids are not physically compromised, their vascular supply may go into spasm and the glands enter a state of temporary or permanent shock making them nonfunctional. The current practice in high-risk cases is to start rT3 and AdcalD3 immediately after operation and to check calcium levels at 8 and 16 h to see if there is a tendency for hypocalcemia. As always, a multidisciplinary team approach involving endocrinologists is advisable.

Key Points

1. Hypercalcemia should be treated by intravenous fluid rehydration and urgent intravenous bisphosphonate administration. The commonest causes are metastatic malignancy and hyperparathyroidism.
2. Diabetic ketoacidosis should be treated by intravenous fluid replacement, intravenous insulin with careful monitoring in a multidisciplinary setting.
3. Diabetic patients being admitted for emergency surgery require intravenous control of their blood glucose irrespective of the severity of their diabetes.
4. Pheochromocytoma, presenting as an emergency, in the absence of previous history is extremely rare. If suspected, surgery should be abandoned pending appropriate treatment and investigation of possible underlying disease.

5. After thyroid or parathyroid surgery, an increasing neck swelling will indicate an impending compartment syndrome due to hemorrhage. The consequence of this is potential airways compromise which can be easily treated by early removal of sutures and evacuation of hematoma if necessary.

6. Bilateral recurrent laryngeal nerve involvement after thyroid or parathyroid surgery may lead to airways compromise through bilateral adduction of the vocal cords or reduction of the airway in an already compromised patient.

7. Thyrotoxic crisis: take electrolytes, glucose, TFTs. a) Give Potassium Iodide (600mg i.v.) then 2g po for less than 2 weeks. b) Prophlthiouracil 300md/day or Carbimazole 30mg TDS po given before Potasium Iodide. c)treat any associated Adrenal failure, Hypoxia, DVT/PE, dialysis, fluid loss, LVF and Hyperpyrexia.

Chapter 4
Trauma and Orthopedic Emergencies

Alan Askari and Jitendra Mangwani

Introduction

Orthopedic emergencies are relatively common and can be associated with a potentially limb- or even life-threatening clinical situation. Patients usually present in distress (often after a sudden event, for example, fall, car accident) and sometimes in chaotic circumstances of the emergency department, making examination and clinical management challenging.

Some patients (such as the "trauma call") may have multiple injuries and will require a multidisciplinary approach to treatment. In all emergencies, it is of vital importance to take a relevant history (if possible), perform a thorough examination, and request appropriate investigations. Time is of essence; in certain conditions, a delay in decision making or treatment may lead to an adverse outcome, for example, a missed compartment syndrome leading to possible loss of limb.

A. Askari, MB ChB, MRCS (Eng) (✉)
Department of Trauma and Orthopaedics,
Colchester Hospital University Foundation NHS Trust, Essex, UK
e-mail: awaskari@hotmail.com

J. Mangwani, M.B.B.S. (GOLD MEDAL), M.S. (ORTH),
FRCS (TR & ORTH)
Department of Trauma and Orthopaedics,
University Hospitals of Leicester, Leicester Royal Infirmary,
Leicester, UK
e-mail: jmangwani@hotmail.com

I. Shergill et al. (eds.), *Surgical Emergencies in Clinical Practice*, 53
DOI 10.1007/978-1-4471-2876-2_4,
© Springer-Verlag London 2013

In the orthopedic patient, it is easy to be distracted by "the fracture" and miss an even bigger injury or condition. The classic example being the elderly "NOF" patient who not so uncommonly sustained the fracture as a result of a collapse due to other pathology (stroke, myocardial infarction, arrhythmia, urinary sepsis, etc.). It is therefore extremely important to have a holistic approach in the management of the trauma patient.

Fractures in children can present a particular challenge both in terms of clinical examination and surgical management. It is important to include parents in the management of children with trauma to help cope with what is understandably an anxious time for them.

Clinical Case Scenario 1: Neck of Femur Fracture

Case Presentation

An 86-year-old lady, who has suffered from osteoporosis for many years, falls in a residential home while going to the bathroom in the middle of the night. She is unable to get up and spends the night on the floor until the warden finds her the following morning as part of a routine visit. In the emergency department, she is dehydrated and lethargic; her right lower limb appears shorter than the left and externally rotated. There is tenderness over the greater trochanter, no active movement is possible, and there is severe pain on attempted passive movement of the right lower limb.

Key Features of History and Examination

Causes

Majority of neck of femur fractures occur in the elderly and are usually traumatic (commonly after a fall from standing). In younger patients, high-energy trauma such as motorbike or vehicle collision is the main cause. In patients with active cancer, pathological neck of femur fractures can occur with minimal or no trauma. Osteoporotic bone is more likely to fracture. In the elderly, during history-taking and examination, it is also important to ascertain any factors *preceding* the trauma, that is, why did the patient fall? Was it a simple mechanical trip, or was there a syncopal episode secondary to cardiac event or an infective process, for example, a urinary tract or lower respiratory tract infection?

Clinical Manifestation

As with any fracture, pain is a common complaint. Pain may be experienced either deep in the groin or down the thigh and into the knee. Inability to weight bear is strongly suspicious of a fracture. Tenderness over the greater trochanter and pain on rolling the hip are common findings. Palpation of the groin may illicit pain. Usually no or minimal movement in the hip (especially straight leg raise) is possible on the affected side. Neurovascular examination should be performed. It is important to always examine the joint below and above any suspected site of pathology. In neck of femur fractures, the lower back and the knee should also be examined.

Principles of Acute Management

Immediate management of associated injuries (i.e., airway, breathing, circulation) takes priority followed by pain relief and IV fluid resuscitation. Blood tests, ECG, and CXR are commonly performed to establish a possible cause, other than direct trauma, as well as preparation for possible anesthetic and surgical treatment.

Discussion

Diagnosis

As with any joint or bone where there is a suspicion of a fracture, X-rays (at least two views 90° to each other) should be performed. Neck of femur fractures can be variable, and their treatment depends on the type and anatomical site of the fracture. The Garden classification is used to categorize different types of fractures.

1. Garden stage I: Incomplete, undisplaced fractures
2. Garden stage II: Complete, undisplaced fractures
3. Garden stage III: Complete fracture, incompletely displaced
4. Garden stage IV: Complete fracture, completely displaced

Treatment and Prognosis

The treatment of the fractures depends on the site of the fracture. The neck of the femur is supplied by three main arteries:

- Medial circumflex artery
- Lateral circumflex artery
- Artery of round ligament of femoral head

The artery of the round ligament supplies the proximal part of the femoral head, while the medial and lateral circumflex arteries anastomose with each other and supply the distal part of the femoral head.

- *Intracapsular fractures*: An intracapsular fracture (i.e., a fracture proximal to the greater and lesser trochanters) usually leads to significant disruption of the blood supply to the femoral head as the anastomosis is disrupted. These fractures have a very high incidence of avascular necrosis. The head of the femur is usually not salvageable and therefore replaced by an artificial implant called a hemiarthroplasty.
- *Extracapsular fractures*: In extracapsular fractures, that is, fractures across the greater and lesser trochanters, the femoral head is usually salvageable (as the medial-lateral circumflex anastomosis is not disrupted). The fracture in

these cases can be managed with a dynamic hip screw (DHS) or intramedullary hip screw (IMHS).

Key Points

1. Neck of femur fractures is common in the elderly usually after a fall and may have other factors precipitating the trauma.
2. Inability to weight bear and pain on rolling the hip are highly suspicious of hip fracture.
3. As with any fracture, at least two X-ray views should be taken.
4. The Garden classification is used to categorize fractures.
5. Displaced intracapsular fractures usually lead to avascular necrosis of the head and require replacement of the head – hemiarthroplasty. Extracapsular fractures are managed with a DHS or IMHS.

Clinical Case Scenario 2: Compartment Syndrome

Case Presentation

A 25-year-old male collided with a white van while riding his motorbike at approximately 45 mph on a wet country road. On arrival in accident and emergency department, his GCS was 15, airway patent, chest clear, abdomen soft, nontender. His observations were stable. He complained of pain and "pins and needles" in the left leg. On examination, he had multiple abrasions on both knees. His right leg was entirely normal, his left leg was swollen, extremely tender; both dorsalis pedis and posterior tibialis pulses were present. An X-ray showed a fracture of left tibia and fibula midshaft.

Key Features of History and Examination

Definition

Compartment syndrome occurs when the tissue pressure of a closed anatomical space (compartment) exceeds the perfusion pressure to that space resulting in tissue ischemia and death.

Causes

Compartment syndrome is commonly caused by fracture within a closed compartment, usually tibial and radial fractures and crush injuries, although it may also occur in purely soft tissue injury such as burns. Application of tight surgical dressing or casts may also precipitate in compartment syndrome.

Clinical Manifestation

The gentleman in the case has signs and symptoms consistent with compartment syndrome. The commonly quoted sign of a pulseless limb is usually a late sign. Classical signs of compartment syndrome are the 5 P's:

- Pain
- Pallor
- Pulselessness
- Paraesthesia
- Paralysis

More commonly, compartment syndrome presents as swelling and extreme or disproportionate pain to injury sustained. Pain on stretching of muscles in the affected compartment is one of the earliest signs. Occasionally, redness and paraesthesia may also be present, but again these may be late manifestations.

Principles of Acute Management

A high index of clinical suspicion is vital for diagnosis. Objectively, compartment pressure measurements can be taken. Measurements can be taken using pressure transducer modules which consist of a needle and an electronic meter. The needle is inserted into the relevant muscle compartment and the meter gives a reading. This reading is subtracted from the diastolic blood pressure of the patient at the time. If the pressure difference between the meter reading and the diastolic blood pressure is less than 30 mmHg, it is an indication of increased pressure in the compartment, and hence the limb is at threat of ischemia. If there is any doubt regarding diagnosis of whether compartment syndrome is present or not, surgical intervention is advocated.

Discussion

Compartment syndrome is an orthopedic emergency that requires immediate surgical decompression in the form of a fasciotomy (cutting of the fascia). The muscle compartment is released on at least two sides using large incisions. If there is necrotic muscle tissue present, it would require debridement. The wound is left open until swelling subsides and closed at a later date. Several trips to theater may be required, and it is not uncommon to debride dead tissues two or three times. Studies have shown that the most important factor determining outcome is the speed of diagnosis. Early diagnosis and intervention is key to better recovery.

Key Points

1. Compartment syndrome occurs when compartment pressure exceeds capillary pressure within that compartment.
2. It is mainly caused by closed fractures, crush injuries, and burns (rarely spontaneous).

3. It is an orthopedic emergency that requires a high index of suspicion.
4. Features are extreme pain, swelling, and redness in affected limb. Pulselessness is a LATE sign.
5. Fasciotomy, debridement, and delayed closure are the treatments.

Clinical Case Scenario 3: Septic Arthritis

Case Presentation

A 4-year-old boy is brought in to the emergency department by his concerned mother. The child has not been his happy self for the last 2 days. He has vomited twice yesterday and is walking with a limp and not playing with his toys. There is no history of injury.

The child has no significant past medical history and has normal childhood milestones. On examination, the patient has a temperature of 37.9 °C, looks flushed, and is walking with a limp, dragging his right hip. The left hip is normal, but the right hip is extremely painful on minimal movement.

Key Features of History and Examination

Definition

Septic arthritis is the invasion of a joint by a pathogenic organism, usually bacterial, although viral and fungal arthritis can also occur.

Causes

The invading pathogen can be transported from other sites of infection already present in the body (lower respiratory tract infection or urinary tract infection) or can be spontaneous and affect any joint. There is increased risk in immunocompromised and diabetic patients.

Clinical Manifestation and Examination

Septic arthritis can occur spontaneously in native joints. The incidence of septic arthritis in the developed world is approximately 1 in 100,000, but a much higher incidence is reported in the developing world (as high as 1 in 5,000 in certain parts of Africa). The most common organism responsible is *Staphylococcus aureus*, followed by *Streptococcus* and *Enterobacter*. As with the examination of any joint, a systematic approach is required: observation, palpation, active movement, and passive movement. Typically, the superficial joints such as knees and elbows are red and inflamed, but these signs may be absent in deeper joints such as hip joints. There may be cellulitic skin changes and tracking of infection up or down the joint. Palpate the joint and look for any swelling or collection of fluid. Feel the overlying skin for warmth. Palpate regional lymph nodes (in this case the inguinal region). The patient will complain of severe pain on the slightest movement of the joint. Passive movement is markedly reduced and very painful. Active movement is usually severely restricted. Check pulses and neurological status of the limb.

Principles of Acute Management

Investigations and Diagnosis

A very high index of suspicion is required, and any joint where there is suspicion of septic arthritis should be aspirated and sent to the laboratory for urgent microscopy, Gram staining, and culture. If infection is chronic, plain film X-rays may show signs of osteomyelitis such as: periosteal elevation, bony destruction (osteolytic lesions), soft tissue swelling, and free gas. Blood cultures should be sent in systemically unwell or pyrexial patients. A high white cell count may be present, but a normal count does not rule out septic arthritis. According to Kocher's criteria, a child who is unable to weight bear with a white cell count of more than 12,000 and an ESR of 40 and a temperature above 37.5 has an almost 97 % of having septic arthritis. Several studies have shown that normal CRP level has a high predictive value for excluding septic arthritis.

Discussion

The definitive treatment of septic arthritis is a combination of broad-spectrum antibiotics and surgical drainage. IV antibiotics should be used in all patients with acute septic arthritis. If patients are medically fit for surgery, joint drainage (open/ arthroscopy) can be performed, and a thorough washout of the joint is essential. Some patients may require more than one washout treatment. In patients who are systemically well, antibiotic therapy should be withheld pending joint aspirate or drainage to obtain a sample. Advice from microbiologists should be sought regarding the appropriate antibiotic regime and length of treatment. A significant proportion of patients have irreversible destruction of the joint despite aggressive treatment. Affected joints run a higher risk of degenerative joint conditions in the future. Some patients will develop long-term sequelae.

Key Points

1. Septic arthritis is the infection of a joint by an organism.
2. Skin abrasions or cuts can increase chances of joint infection, especially in immunocompromised or diabetic patients.
3. It is characterized by marked reduction in joint mobility and pain.

4. Needle aspiration should be carried out on any joint suspected of infection.
5. Treatment involves surgical washout and aggressive antibiotic therapy.

Clinical Case Scenario 4: Supracondylar Fracture of Humerus

Case Scenario

A 6-year-old boy has a fall from "monkey bars" at a local playground. The child complains of severe pain in the left elbow and will not permit movement. On examination, the child is in great distress, and the left elbow appears deformed. The patient reports pins and needles over the entire hand but particularly over the volar aspect of the radial three digits. Capillary refill in the fingernail beds is 4 s. After careful examination, the child does not have any other injuries.

Key Features of History and Examination

Definition and Types

Supracondylar humerus fracture is a common injury in children, typically affecting 5–7-year-olds.
They are usually sustained after a fall from height (e.g., monkey bars, trampolines, and bouncy castles). In majority of cases, it is the nondominant side that is affected. They are divided into *extension* and *flexion* types depending on which plane the distal fragment of the fracture moves, posterior or anterior, respectively.

- *Extension type*: Also known as *posterior* fractures. They comprise of 97 % of supracondylar humerus fractures. The distal part of the fracture moves backward (posteriorly) usually due to fall onto an outstretched hand with the elbow in full extension. The modified *Gartland* classification is used to describe the fracture types:

- *Type I*: A nondisplaced or minimally displaced (less than 2 mm) fracture. This type of fracture is very stable and is treated conservatively.
- *Type II*: Fracture is displaced by more than 2 mm, and the posterior cortex is hinged, that is, there is discontinuity of the anterior humerus. This type of fracture requires surgical intervention.
- *Type III*: These fractures are characteristically completely displaced. There may be rotational deformity and neurovascular compromise.

- *Flexion type*: Also known as *anterior* fractures due to the anterior displacement of the distal part of the fracture.

They are rare and only make up a small minority (1–3 %) of supracondylar fractures. They can cause ulnar nerve injury.

Examination and Diagnosis

With any acute injury (especially in children), it is important to take the state of the whole patient into account and not be distracted by an obvious fracture, deformity, or dislocation and miss an even bigger, more subtle, injury. The patient's general well-being, GCS, and demeanor should be noted. Any obvious thoracic or abdominal pathology should be ruled out. A systematic approach to the skeletal system should be undertaken. One should be mindful of potential nonaccidental injury. With regard to assessing limb fractures, the following should be noted:

- *Deformity*: Compare limbs on both sides, and look for any deformity. Deformities may be obvious or very subtle; obvious ones will most likely have a fracture.
- *Skin*: Look for telltale signs – is the skin intact or has it been broken? If broken, has it been broken by an underlying fracture (open fracture)?

- *Neurovascular status*: Check the presence, quality, and strength of both radial and ulnar pulses. Assess and record the capillary refill in the nail beds. A delayed refill is a sign of significant vascular compromise. Check sensation and motor function distal to the fracture (moving fingers etc.), and look for sensory changes, that is, feelings of "pins and needles."
- *Movement*: Is there any movement at the elbow? If the patient will not permit any movement, they should not be forced to do so.

Diagnosis is made on plain X-ray. A fracture may be clearly seen on an X-ray; if not, look for subtle "telltale" signs such as elevation of the fat pads around the elbow. Describe and record the fracture seen clearly, that is, the site of the fracture, degree of displacement, presence of fat pad, closed/open.

Principles of Acute Management

The aim is to restore the fracture to its anatomical position (reduction) and keep it in the correct position (immobilization) until such time that significant healing has taken place. Treatment of supracondylar fractures depends on the severity of displacement.

- Gartland type I: Since these fractures are nondisplaced, they are treated conservatively (with above-elbow back slab with the elbow at 90° flexion). The period of immobilization is dependent on the age of the child
- Gartland type II: Type II fractures require manipulation under a general anesthetic to restore them to the normal anatomical position. The fracture is reduced in operating theater and screened using X-rays. If the fracture looks stable and not likely to displace, a back slab is used to hold it in place. If the fracture appears unstable and likely to displace, Kirschner wires (K-wires) are used to hold the fracture in place. The wires can be taken out at a later date (usually 4 weeks), by which time the fracture should have formed a callus and healing should be well underway.
- Gartland type III: These fractures are likely to displace unless fixed with K-wires. In some instances, the fracture may require ORIF (open reduction internal fixation). This

involves making an incision over the fracture, opening the fracture, and restoring the anatomical position (open reduction), and fixation with K-wires (internal fixation) to keep it in place.

- Flexion fractures: The treatment for flexion (anterior) fractures is similar to extension fractures and also depends on the degree of displacement. Undisplaced fractures are treated nonsurgically. Minor displacements would require manipulation $\pm$ K-wire, and major displacements require manipulation and K-wire or ORIF.

Discussion

In this particular example, there are signs of neurovascular compromise, increased capillary refill time, and "pins and needles." These findings warrant urgent treatment of the injury. They require prompt assessment and accurate documentation of clinical findings. Orthopedic seniors and vascular surgeons should be made aware of such cases early. In majority of cases, the blood supply and sensation improve quickly after the fracture is reduced to its original anatomical position. In cases where the radial and ulnar pulses are compromised, the fracture is reduced and the pulses are checked. If the pulse has returned and is of good strength and the capillary refill has returned to normal, the fracture can be fixed. If the pulses have failed to return, the fracture is not to be fixed until vascular surgeons have explored vessels and a blood supply has been re-established.

Key Points

1. Supracondylar fractures are common in children and are of two types: extension and flexion.
2. A full examination of the patient as well as assessment of the neurovascular status of the limb must be carried out.
3. The modified Gartland system is used to categorize fractures.

4. Nondisplaced (type I) fractures are treated conservatively, whereas displaced fractures (type II and III fractures) require manipulation (closed/open) and fixation with K-wires.
5. Pulseless fractures are emergencies that may require the input of vascular surgeons as well as orthopedics.

Clinical Case Scenario 5: Poly-Trauma Patient

Case Presentation

A 21-year-old male motorcyclist is brought into the emergency department's resuscitation room after he had a head-on collision with a van at 50 mph. The patient was wearing a helmet and protective clothing. He is brought in on a spinal board and is in a hard collar. His GCS (Glasgow Coma Score) is 15. He is complaining of neck, lower abdomen, and hip pain. He is tachycardic and hypotensive. He has bruising over his lower abdomen and has a pelvic binder in place.

Key Features of History and Examination and Principles of Acute Management

Trauma patients may have multiple injuries; therefore, a thorough and systematic method of assessment is required to prevent important diagnoses being overlooked. To this end, an internationally recognized protocol is in place called ATLS (Adult Trauma Life Support) which involves a team of different specialties working together quickly to assess and treat trauma patients. These specialties include emergency medicine, anesthetics, general surgeons, and orthopedics. If pregnant women or children are involved, obstetric, gynecology, and pediatric teams form part of the trauma team.

The ATLS pathway is a logical step-by-step method of identifying and treating pathology in trauma patients. The pathway is split into *primary* and *secondary* surveys.

Primary Survey

- *A – Airway* and *C-spine immobilization*: Check the airway for any signs of obstruction; look for any bruising over the trachea. Is the patient maintaining their own airway? If they are talking, it is safe to assume they are maintaining their own airway. If the airway is compromised (either due to direct trauma to the neck, jaw, or face or indirectly as a result of low GCS), it needs to be secured. Simple airway maneuvers such as chin lift and jaw thurst can be performed. A definitive airway via endotracheal intubation or emergency tracheostoty may need to be established. Part of "A" is "triple immobilization" of the cervical spine, that is, hard collar, cervical blocks, and tape.
- *B – Breathing*: Expose the patient's chest; look for any obvious deformity or bruising over the chest. Is there any tenderness over the ribs? Is breathing normal or "paradoxical," that is, the chest caving in as the patient breathes in (normally the thorax should swing out)? If there is caving, the patient may have multiple rib fractures with a "flail segment." Is the chest normal to percussion? Normally, the lungs are filled with air and should be resonant. Dullness to percussion indicates a possible hemothorax or lung collapse. Is there equal air entry on auscultation? In penetrating chest wounds, tension pneumothorax could quickly develop. This may require urgent treatment in the form of a chest drain with underwater seal or, if immediately life threatening, a needle decompression in the second intercostals space. Oxygen saturation and respiratory rate should be carefully documented and routinely checked.
- *C – Circulation*: Does the patient appear shut down/pale? Measure blood pressure and heart rate. Tachycardia may be due to pain, but when coupled with hypotension, it is a worrying sign. Always think bleeding as "1 on the floor and 4 more" parts of the body. The "1 on the floor" refers to any open wounds that are visibly bleeding. If this is the case, maintain direct and constant pressure over the bleed. The "4 more" part refers to the four main body parts that trauma patients tend to bleed from: chest, abdomen, pelvis,

and long bones (especially femur). These four parts need to be checked carefully. Listen to the chest for signs of hemopneumothorax. "Muffling of heart sounds" in blunt trauma to the chest (i.e., a driver's chest striking the steering wheel) and hemodynamic instability are signs of cardiac tamponade which may require pericardiocentesis. Observe the abdomen for signs of bruising and palpate for tenderness. The spleen is the most commonly injured organ in blunt trauma with potentially torrential blood loss. Hepatic and renal trauma can also result in significant blood loss. The abdomen can distend to accommodate a large quantity of blood. The pelvis can fracture in several ways, the most serious of which are "open book" and "vertical shearing fractures." If there is clear deformity or potentially a pelvic fracture, the pelvis should be "bound" by a pelvic binder or, if none available, bed sheets or towels. The long bones especially the femur can bleed significantly. Look for deformities and palpate the long bones carefully.

- *D – Disability*: Assessment of the patient's neurological status. Any abnormality in sensation or deficit in movement may be due to spinal trauma. The Glasgow Coma Scale (GCS) is a useful tool in assessing the patient's neurological status. Examine the pupils, looking for symmetry, and note their reaction to light. Asymmetrical pupils may be the only signs of serious intracranial pathology.
- *E – Exposure*: Expose the patient fully (while avoiding hypothermia) and look for other overt signs of injury.
- *DEFG*: "*Don't Ever Forget Glucose*": Measure blood glucose level. Hypoglycemia should be corrected.

Secondary Survey

The patient is log rolled (with an experienced clinician stabilizing the head), and a thorough examination of the back is performed, looking for obvious signs of injury (bruising, laceration, deformity). The vertebrae are palpated for tenderness. A PR exam is performed and the patient is asked to squeeze against a finger to rule out signs of spinal cord damage. Blood per rectum may be a sign of significant pelvic injury. The patient is systematically assessed from head to toe for injuries (lacerations, contusions, skin tears, fractures of small bones).

Investigations: A standard "trauma series" of plain radiographs should be performed on trauma patients. This includes:

- C-spine: Look for vertebral alignment, fractures.
- Chest: Look for hemothorax, pneumothorax, fractured ribs (fractures of the first and second rib indicate significant force applied to the thorax).
- Pelvis: Look for pelvic and neck of femur fractures.
- Other X-rays: Of any relevant part of the body found to have injury on secondary survey.
- ECG: All trauma patients should have an ECG, looking for ECG changes that may arise secondary to chest trauma.
- Blood tests: FBC, U&E, LFT, amylase, clotting, group, and save.
- Arterial blood gas: In hypoxic or hemodynamically compromised patients.
- CT: CT imaging may be required for any part of the body: head, C-spine, chest, abdomen, and pelvis. Sometimes, whole body CT is required in unconscious patients.

Discussion

Treatment depends on the type and severity of injury. Clearing the C-spine on both clinical and radiological examination is important. Trauma patients may require little more than overnight observation (in some instances, patients can go home same day if there is no clinical evidence of injury and investigations are normal). Equally, trauma patients may need significant input from multiple specialties such as general surgery, orthopedics, plastics, vascular, neurosurgery, intensive care/anesthetics, pediatrics, obstetrics, and gynecology. In some instances, an emergency life-saving operation (laparotomy, splenectomy, external fixation of hip fractures, etc.) may be required. Prognosis and length of hospital stay are extremely variable depending on the extent of injuries sustained. In some patients, urgent transfer to a relevant unit may be needed.

Key Points

1. Trauma patients require multispecialty input.
2. A systematic and competent approach (primary and secondary survey) is vital to quickly assess and treat patients and to ensure that no injuries are missed.
3. Injuries should be treated as they are identified.
4. The extent of injuries and treatments required can be extremely variable.
5. Hospital stay and prognosis depends on the extent of injuries and treatments required.

Chapter 5
ENT Emergencies

Krishnam Penumetcha, Waseem Jerjes, N. Patel, and Tahwinder Upile

Introduction

Many ENT emergencies are common surgical presentations which can be simply and effectively managed at a junior surgical stage. They are also within the remit of general and emergency surgeons in host institutions where ENT as a specialty is not immediately available.

Many undergraduate curricula do not include otorhinolaryngology and now reserve ENT teaching for postgraduate students leaving many deficits for the trainee surgeon. An

K. Penumetcha, MRCS, DO HNS, M.S (Otolaryngology) •
W. Jerjes, B.Sc. (hons), Ph.D., M.Sc., B.D.S., M.B.B.S.
Department of ENT, Barnet and Chase Farm Hospitals,
Enfield, Greater London, UK
e-mail: drkrispen@yahoo.com

N. Patel, FRCS
Head and Neck Unit, Department of ENT,
Southampton University Hospitals, Southampton, UK

T. Upile, B.Sc. (hons), M.Sc., M.S., M.D., FRCS (Gen Surg), FRCS
(OTO), FRCS (ORL-HNS), DFFP, FHEA, MRCGP
Department of ENT, Barnet and Chase Farm Hospitals,
Enfield, Greater London, UK

Head and Neck Unit, University College London Hospitals,
Greater London, UK

I. Shergill et al. (eds.), *Surgical Emergencies in Clinical Practice*,   73
DOI 10.1007/978-1-4471-2876-2_5,
© Springer-Verlag London 2013

understanding of surgical airways management is imperative for anyone dealing with acute referrals and trauma patients. The use of transtracheal catheters (Grey/Brown Venflon), or in some instances laryngeal mask, remains a valuable airways adjunct in an emergency. It should also be noted that often ENT hemorrhage is trivialized as a simple epistaxis, but caution must be exercised and where appropriate ATLS principles adhered to. Comorbidity must also be noted so that the treatment initiation thresholds are lowered in cadiovascularly compromised individuals.

It is essential that multidisciplinary care is entered into early, and that when required, appropriate referral is made at the opportune time to more senior and/or specialist teams. We have selected the cases based upon their frequency of presentation, need for correct initial management, and due to the medicolegal consequences of poor management.

Clinical Case Scenario 1: Epistaxis (Nose Bleed)

Case Presentation

A 54-year-old male patient presented to the casualty with 1 h history of spontaneous, intermittent, but profuse nose bleeds. Patient is a known hypertensive and takes aspirin daily. This is his first presentation and is accompanied by his wife who is extremely anxious and worried. He is able to give a full history himself and allows observations by the triage nurse who informs you that he is hemodynamically stable.

Key Features in the History and Examination

Various factors need to be established in the history: Was the epistaxis spontaneous or traumatic? How often and how long? Were there any contributory factors (see common causes of nose bleeds in discussion)? Bleeding tendencies in the family? Current medication: anticoagulants, antiplatelets – aspirin/clopidogrel – anti-hypertensives, etc.

Examination

Good light source, nasal specula, and suction are essential for thorough examination. Best examined in sitting position on a couch. Assess the side and site of nose bleed, that is, left or right, anterior or posterior bleeding. Assess blood loss, check pulse and blood pressure.

Investigations

Gain IV access and set up IV fluids. Take blood for full blood counts, coagulation profile (INR in warfarin users), and group and save.

Principles of Acute Management

Initially, consider ATLS pathway for acute hemorrhage, even if the amount looks trivial.

First Aid

In the event of an active nose bleed, sit the patient on a couch and advise to pinch the soft anterior part of the nose firmly (NOT over the bony part) for at least 10 min. Lean forward and spit any blood running down the throat to avoid swallowing/aspiration. Place an icepack over nasal bridge.

Nasal Cautery

Nasal cautery can be attempted if the bleeding point is anterior and visible. Avoid using silver nitrate if the nose is actively bleeding. Prior to attempting nasal cautery, pack a piece cotton wool, dental roll soaked in Xylocaine with adrenaline solution over the area to be cauterized for a few minutes. Touch the mucosa around the bleeding point in a circle to allow any feeding blood vessels cauterized first before attempting the cautery of main bleeding vessel. Silver nitrate is dabbed over the bleeding point for 1 or 2 s at a time. Indiscriminate use of silver nitrate/electrocautery can cause septal perforation/ unintentional burns.

Nasal Packing

For anterior nasal packing, Merocel tampon is preferred. To insert the tampon, lift the tip of the nose and slide the lubricated tampon along the floor of nose (NOT toward the top of the head). This tampon is made of polyvinyl alcohol sponge which when hydrated with water or saline expands in the nasal cavity and arrests bleeding by pressure effect. The Merocel tampon should be removed from the nasal cavity within 48 h. BIPP (bismuth iodoform paraffin paste) ribbon pack is an alternative but needs skill, good light source, and appropriate instruments for effective packing.

For posterior nose bleeds, a variety of balloons are available. The Brighton epistaxis balloons have two ports to inflate the posterior and anterior balloons which sit in the postnasal space and in the nasal cavity, respectively. The Foley urinary catheter is a useful alternative. It is passed into the nasopharynx, inflated and pulled anteriorly to snugly fit the posterior choana. It needs to be secured anteriorly with umbilical clamp to prevent slipping back. It is important to put padding between the clamp and nose to prevent pressure damage to the skin of nose. Rarely, profuse and uncontrolled posterior nasal bleeds need examination under general anesthetic and endoscopic ligation of the sphenopalatine artery.

When treating the epistaxis, always address the underlying cause for a successful management. For example, in patients using anticoagulants always check the reason for anticoagulant use. Advice from the hematologist may be required in reversing the anticoagulant effects.

Discussion

Epistaxis (nose bleed) is a common ENT problem. It varies from minor to life-threatening emergency. Any age group can be affected, but it is much more common in children and the elderly. The anterior part of the nasal septum (Littles's area) is the usual site of bleeding owing to its rich blood supply. Majority of the nose bleeds are minor and self-limiting.

Common causes of epistaxis are as follows:

Local
> Trauma – blunt injury or nose picking (digital trauma)
> Dry mucosa and crusting (central heating, deviated nasal septum, hot weather)
> Idiopathic
> Tumors in the nose
> Iatrogenic

Systemic
> Hypertension
> Coagulation disorders/use of anticoagulants
> Hereditary hemorrhagic telangiectasia (Osler-Weber-Rendu disease) – an autosomal dominant inherited condition where weakness of capillary walls leads to hemangiomas that bleed.

Clinical Case Scenario 2:
Periorbital Cellulitis and Acute Sinusitis

Periorbital Cellulitis

Case Presentation

A 6-year-old boy presented with a 2 day history of progressive swelling of left upper eyelid and periorbital region, following a recent common cold. He was unable to open his eyes and complains of pain. He was also noted to have mild fever since 1 day.

Key Features in the History and Examination

A complication of acute ethmoidal sinusitis. More common in children. In the early stages, the infection is confined to the eyelid and periorbital area only. The infection can spread rapidly to the eye or retrobulbar structures and can cause permanent loss of vision in a matter of hours.

Typical Presentation:
> History of recent URTI ± nasal discharge
> Pain, tenderness, and swelling around the eye (usually upper eyelid swelling prominent)
> Difficulty in opening the eye

Warning Signs (Indicating Spread of Infection to the Orbit)

> Conjunctival congestion
> Proptosis/diplopia
> Change in color vision (one of the early signs; red is the first to be affected)
> Pain on eye movement or reduced range of eye movement
> Change in visual acuity
> Abnormal afferent papillary light reflexes in the affected eye
> Intracranial complications – persistent headache, nausea, vomiting, pyrexia, altered consciousness

Principles of Acute Management

Treatment should be aimed at the underlying sinusitis. High index of suspicion, early diagnosis, and input from ENT and ophthalmology are all essential in managing this condition.

Treat with broad-spectrum IV antibiotics (e.g., Augmentin), nasal decongestants, and analgesics.

CT scans of sinuses, i.e. coronal views of paranasal sinuses and axial views through orbits, should be obtained if there is any suspicion of orbital involvement. Intra-orbital abscess requires urgent surgical intervention.

When managing conservatively, frequent eye checks are essential.

Acute Sinusitis

Often follows URTI. Acute exacerbations of chronic sinusitis are common.

Presentation

> Nasal congestion and purulent discharge
> Facial pain particularly over maxillae/cheeks
> Pyrexia
> Swelling of the face uncommon
> Visual disturbances not a feature of uncomplicated acute sinusitis

Treatment

> Nasal decongestant, for example, Xylometazoline spray
> Analgesia
> Broad-spectrum oral antibiotics like Augmentin or Ciprofloxacin (common infective agents – *Streptococcus pneumoniae, Haemophilus influenza, Moraxella catarrhalis, and Staphylococcus aureus*)
> Generally do not require admission

Acute Throat Infections

Acute Tonsillitis

Case Scenario

An 18-year-old young lady presented to the emergency department with a 3-day history of persistent sore throat, high fever, and inability to swallow due to pain (Fig. 5.1).

Key Features of History and Examination

> Sore throat, pain, and difficulty on swallowing
> Past history of sore throats/tonsillitis

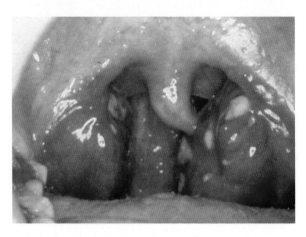

FIGURE 5.1 An intraoral view of erythematous tonsils with debris in the swollen crypts. Follicular tonsillitis

Referred otalgia

Fever and malaise

Bad breath

On examination – enlarged congested tonsils ± white exudates on tonsils; palpable and sometimes tender cervical lymphadenopathy

In the early stages, glandular fever is often hard to distinguish from acute bacterial tonsillitis.

Principles of Acute Management

Analgesia, antibiotics, and maintain hydration.

Oral or IV antibiotics depending on patient's general state.

Penicillin V/clarithromycin are the preferred oral antibiotics. Amoxicillin is best avoided in suspected glandular fever because it can cause severe skin rash.

Often patients have difficulty in swallowing. Anesthetic gargles temporarily relieve the odynophagia. Soluble oral or rectally administered analgesia is preferable.

Patients who are unable to swallow fluids adequately will require hospital admission for IV antibiotics, analgesics, and IV hydration.

Investigations: FBC, U&E, glandular fever screening test, LFTs (if glandular fever suspected) and throat swab.

In patients with glandular fever one or two doses IV steroid injections (dexamethasone 8 mg) can give significant symptomatic relief.

General Discussion

Acute tonsillitis is a common ENT problem seen in emergency department and general practice. Tonsillitis can affect any age group but is most common in young children and teenagers. Common organisms causing acute bacterial tonsillitis are *Streptococcus* species, *H. influenza,* and *S. aureus.*

Viral tonsillitis is also common but glandular fever (caused by EB virus) deserves special attention owing to the severity of the symptoms and the prolonged course of infection and the sequel.

Glandular fever (*infectious mononucleosis*) is caused by Epstein-Barr virus. It is common in teenagers and young adults. It is usually a self-limiting condition, but the symptoms of tonsillitis are more severe and prolonged. Marked cervical lymphadenopathy (hence the name glandular fever) and occasional hepatosplenomegaly occur in this condition. Diagnosis is confirmed by Monospot or Paul-Bunnell blood test.

Complications of Acute Tonsillitis

Quincy (Peritonsillar Abscess)

Quincy denotes formation of an abscess in the peritonsillar tissue in the soft palate, displacing the uvula to the opposite side. It is almost always unilateral. Patient presents with trismus and drooling of saliva due to inability to swallow.

Aspiration of abscess with a wide bore needle or incision and drainage along with analgesics and IV antibiotics is the mainstay of the treatment. Local anesthetic spray is not generally required. The point where an imaginary line along free edge of anterior tonsillar pillar joins another imaginary line along base of uvula would be the ideal site for aspiration/I&D.

Further aspirations may be required in the following 24–48 h as abscess is likely to recur.

Parapharyngeal Abscess

It can occur as a rare complication of acute tonsillitis. It is more common in immunocompromised patients and in patients with indiscriminate use of steroids for acute tonsillitis (often symptoms are masked). It can be a result of spread of infection into parapharyngeal space or a result of lymph node suppuration. It usually presents with diffuse swelling in the neck or in the lateral pharyngeal wall. Early assessment of airway is important. Patients will need ultrasound examination of neck to locate the site and size of abscess. Treatment includes broad-spectrum IV antibiotics with anaerobic cover and drainage of the abscess (usually external approach required).

Acute Airway Obstruction

Rare complication can occur as a result of significant enlargement of tonsils/adenoids in glandular fever. Patient may develop severe sleep apnea. IV steroids can resolve the airway obstruction dramatically.

Miscellaneous Throat Infections

Acute Pharyngitis

This is a common and self-limiting problem. Patient presents with sore throat and irritation. Dysphagia is rare. Voice is unaffected. On examination, congested/inflamed pharyngeal mucosa is identified.

Principles of Management

Need simple remedies – analgesia and rehydration. Saline/anesthetic gargles give symptomatic relief.

Rarely antibiotics are needed. Admission not required unless dysphagia/odynophagia significant.

Acute Laryngitis

This is a common and self-limiting problem. Inflammation of larynx can occur in isolation or in conjunction with URTI. Noninfective causes include voice abuse and acid reflux.

Patient presents with sore throat, pain on speaking or swallowing, hoarseness of voice/loss of voice, and occasionally cough.

Principles of Management

Reassurance, voice rest, analgesics, and cough suppressants. *Avoid gargling or whispering as both can aggravate laryngitis.*

Ludwig's Angina

This is an uncommon but potentially life threatening infection of the floor of mouth, which usually results from a dental infection. It is more common in adults. *It can cause acute airway problem by upward and backward displacement of tongue due to swelling/abscess in floor of mouth tissues.*

Patient presents with trismus, drooling, dysphagia, and high fever. Bimanual palpation of floor of mouth confirms firm thickening of tissues.

Principles of Management

Treat the infection with high dose IV broad-spectrum antibiotics and maintain IV hydration. If airway problem is imminent, secure airway with nasopharyngeal intubation or tracheostomy, if necessary (Fig. 5.2).

Stridor

Case Scenario

A 3-year-old child was brought to the emergency department with noisy breathing, drooling saliva, and high fever. The child was unable to lie flat and was noted to be sitting forward and using accessory muscles of respiration.

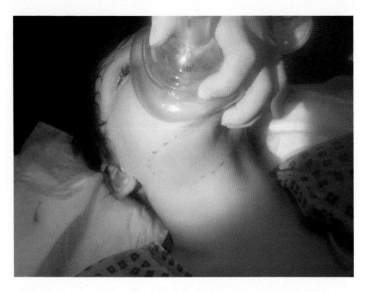

FIGURE 5.2 A young male who presented with progressive subman-dibular swelling from infection causing airways compromise

Key Features of History and Examination

Epiglottitis and Supraglottitis

Acute inflammation of epiglottis and supraglottic structures is a serious condition occurring in children between the ages of 1–5 years, caused by *H. influenza* type B bacteria. It can lead to airway obstruction very rapidly. Since the routine HIB vaccination, this condition is less commonly seen in children in developed countries. Adults are more commonly affected these days and often present with supraglottitis.

Preceding URTI, high temperature muffled voice and rapid onset of stridor indicate possible epiglottitis. *Do not attempt to examine the throat and do not distress the child for IV access*, as this may aggravate the stridor and cause complete airway obstruction. When the diagnosis of epiglottitis is certain, X-raying would be a waste of time, as it does not provide further information. Summon the senior anesthetist and ENT surgeon on call. If the child tolerates, give oxygen by mask and nebulized adrenaline (4 ml of 1 in 10,000) to reduce the edema. Patient is moved to the operating theater at the earliest where airway is best secured by endotracheal intubation, and when this fails, emergency tracheostomy may be necessary.

Discussion

Stridor – high-pitched noise produced by obstructed airway.

Inspiratory stridor – obstruction at the level of vocal cords or above (supraglottic obstruction)

Expiratory stridor – indicates bronchial (wheeze) or tracheal obstruction

Biphasic stridor – stridor on both inspiration and expiration; occurs in subglottic obstruction

Stertor – low-pitched noise produced by pharyngeal airways compromise

Congenital Causes of Stridor

Laryngomalacia
Subglottic stenosis
Glottic web
Bilateral vocal cord palsy

Acquired Causes of Stridor

Foreign body
Infective – epiglottitis/supraglottitis, croup
External trauma
Laryngeal papillomatosis
Angioedema
Laryngeal cancer
Iatrogenic – damage to recurrent laryngeal nerves from thyroid surgery
Subglottic stenosis from prolonged intubation

Other Causes of Stridor

Croup (Acute Laryngo-Tracheo-Bronchitis)

This commonly affects children and involves the whole of upper respiratory tract. It is usually viral in origin but can occur as a result of *H. influenza* infection. Patient presents with history of fever, malaise, muffled voice, barking cough, and occasional stridor. Progression of symptoms is slower than in epiglottitis. In terms of airway obstruction, this condition is less serious than epiglottitis, but on rare occasions can be life threatening.

Principles of Management

Hospital admission for observation, IV antibiotics, IV steroids, and adrenaline nebulizations and ventilatory support where appropriate.

Angioedema (Angioneurotic Edema/Quincke Edema)

This is an allergic reaction leading to swelling of lips, tongue, uvula, or supraglottic structures. Certain food allergies (seafood and nuts), insect stings, or medication can precipitate angioedema. In adults, use of ACE inhibitors (particularly lisinopril) is strongly associated with this condition. The generalized swelling of tongue or supraglottic tissues can compromise the airway rapidly.

Hereditary angioedema is a condition cased by reduced levels or function of C1 esterase inhibitor enzyme causing recurrent episodes of angioedema (Fig. 5.3).

Principles of Management

Medical management with IV steroids and adrenaline nebulizations rapidly resolves the edema. The use of oral steroids and antihistamines is advised further 48–72 h.

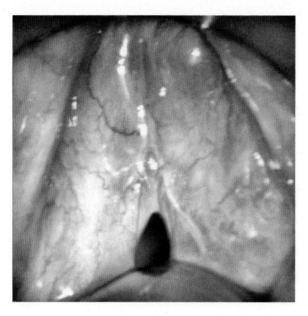

FIGURE 5.3 An endoscopic view of the larynx in angioedema. Note the reduced airway

Foreign Bodies in the Ear, Nose, and Throat Practice

Esophageal Foreign Bodies

Case Scenario

A 50-year-old man presented to the casualty with history of meat bolus stuck in throat while eating steak several hours ago. He thinks there is a piece of bone in the meat. He complains of inability to swallow and keeps spitting saliva.

The cricopharyngeal sphincter is the narrowest part of the esophagus (approximate diameter 12 mm in an adult) and often the site of food bolus impaction. Most foreign bodies pass down harmlessly, but sharp foreign bodies carry a high risk of perforation. Common foreign bodies in esophagus include food bolus, fish bones, poultry, meat bones, coins, and dentures. Complications from esophageal foreign bodies include mediastinitis, airway obstruction, stricture formation, and rarely tracheoesophageal fistula.

Key Features of History and Examination

Symptoms

> Acute onset of partial or complete dysphagia within hours.
> Drooling or spitting of saliva.
> Feeling of obstruction and pain in the lower throat.
> Retrosternal or back pain (interscapular pain) if the FB is stuck at mid-esophagus.
> Chocking spells or stridor are rare but need urgent attention as they indicate potential airway obstruction.
> Fiber-optic nasolaryngoscopy shows pooling of saliva, and on rare occasion the FB may be visualized.

Plain X-ray lateral and AP views of the soft tissues of neck:

Plain X-ray may show the foreign body but cannot exclude one. Cricoid, thyroid, and arytenoids cartilages are often mistaken for FBs and not all foreign bodies are radioopaque. So look for soft tissue swelling in addition to radioopaque object at the level of C5-C6. The only evidence of FB may be air in the upper esophagus on the lateral view of neck. Prevertebral air shadow or surgical emphysema indicates esophageal perforation (Figs. 5.4 and 5.5).

Principles of Acute Management

A good history is essential to establish the type of foreign body ingested. If there is any suggestion of sharp foreign body or bone in esophagus, an urgent endoscopic removal under GA is mandatory.

If the foreign body is a button battery, immediate removal is advised as it can leak causing considerable damage to esophagus.

Soft food bolus impactions are managed conservatively. Patients require hospital admission for observation and IV

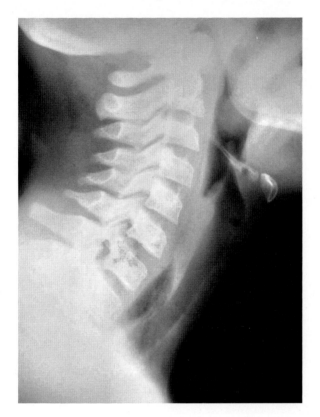

FIGURE 5.4 A lateral soft tissues neck CX-ray showing air in the esophagus

fluids. Injection of smooth muscle relaxant Buscopan (scopolamine) 20 mg IV repeated 8 hourly along with a stat dose of diazepam 10 mg aid in the passage of food bolus to stomach. Trial of fizzy drinks (Coke) help disimpaction on occasions.

If the food bolus fails to pass down within 24 h since ingestion, endoscopic removal under GA is necessary.

Foreign Body: Throat

Common foreign bodies in throat are fish bones and occasionally fragments of chicken bones. Usual sites of lodgement are

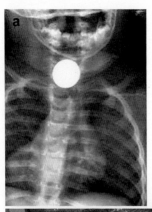

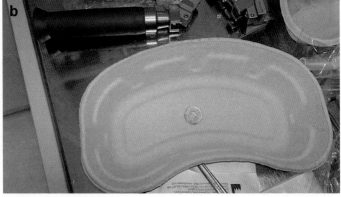

FIGURE 5.5 (a) A plain X-ray chest with an obvious foreign body (a UK 1 pence coin) lodged at the level of the cricopharynx due to muscle spasm and small diameter of the esophagus. (b) The removed foreign body

base of tongue, vallecula, tonsillar fossae, and pyriform sinuses. Patient complains of foreign body sensation and pain in throat and often able to localize. Laryngeal crepitus (rocking of larynx side to side over the cervical vertebral bodies) causes pain. Good head light, tongue depressors, and fiber-optic laryngoscope are useful equipment for visualization of FB. X-ray lateral view of neck reveals radioopaque FBs.

If the foreign body can be visualized, a Magill forceps is a good instrument for removal. Rigid laryngopharyngoscopic examination under GA may be required in some instances for FB removal.

Foreign Body: Bronchus

Foreign bodies can present as airway emergencies. Larger foreign bodies obstructing the upper airway are often expelled (usually by *Heimlich maneuver*) by the time patient comes to the emergency department; otherwise the patient is brought dead and resuscitation would not be possible. Foreign bodies impacted in laryngeal inlet need to removed by direct rigid laryngoscopy with Magill forceps.

Children often aspirate peanuts (most common) and small objects into their bronchus. These children often present with episodes of chocking initially, unexplained cough, unilateral wheeze, and pneumonia. Always think of foreign body aspiration in young children presenting with unexplained cough and pneumonia (*All that wheezes is not Asthma*!). Plain X-rays of chest may show radioopaque FB or lung changes. Removal of FB with operative bronchoscope is the treatment of choice.

Foreign Body: Nose

This is common in children under the age of 3 years. Potential risk of aspiration makes them a relative emergency. Go by the history, as foreign body in the nose is not always visible unless anterior. Unilateral foul smelling bloody discharge from affected nostril may be late presentation of nasal FB. An otoscope, good head light, blunt wax hook, Jobson probe, Tilley's dressing forceps and suction are essential equipment.

Principles of Management

You are likely to get only one chance to remove nasal foreign body, even with a cooperative child. Use wax hook or blunt end of Jobson Horne probe to go beyond the solid foreign body and gently push it outside. For soft and soggy foreign bodies, suction is useful. Forceps are sometimes useful for flat, soft foreign bodies.

An examination under GA may be necessary if the FB cannot be removed, the child is uncooperative, or despite a convincing history the FB is not visualized.

Foreign Body: Ear

Children often put foreign bodies like beads, bits of crayon, paper, small stones, etc., in the ear canal. It is not an absolute emergency and can normally be dealt in civilized hours. A good head light, otoscope, wax hook, suction, and crocodile forceps are essential instruments. Microscope can be useful in some instances. Children usually allow only one attempt at removal. If the child is uncooperative, the FB is best removed under general anesthetic (Fig. 5.6).

Live insects in the ear canal should be killed by drowning in oil before attempting removal. Antihistamines reduce the irritation and itching in ear canal.

Foreign bodies can cause otitis externa, and, therefore, following the removal if bleeding or discharge is noted, topical antibiotic ear drops must be prescribed for a few days.

Traumatic Perforation of Eardrum

It can occur as a result of foreign body in the ear, direct injury, or barotrauma. On examination, the perforation often appears linear and irregular. Do not attempt to clean the blood/clots from the ear. Traumatic perforations almost always heal spontaneously, especially if the patient is young.

Principles of Management

Reassure and advise patient to keep the ears dry. Avoid topical antibiotic ear drops. Prophylactic oral antibiotics are

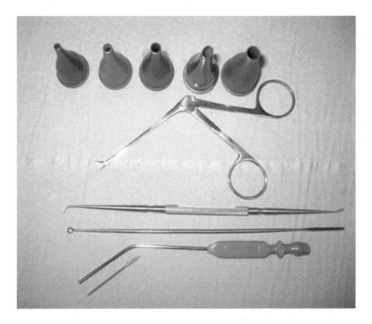

FIGURE 5.6 A low-cost set for the treatment of simple ENT emergencies

prescribed only if the injury is caused by a dirty object. Patients will need an ENT outpatient clinic appointment after 4 weeks for inspection and hearing test.

Acute Ear Infections and Mastoiditis

Otitis Externa

Inflammation of skin of outer ear canal with or without Infection. It is a very common ENT condition presenting to the emergency departments. Patients present with itching, severe throbbing earache, ear discharge, and reduced hearing. In severe cases, patients develop perichondritis of pinna, cellulitis over the face, and fever. On examination, the skin of the ear canal appears swollen and inflamed, and the ear canal appears narrowed, often with scanty purulent discharge.

Furunculosis is a staphylococcal infection of the hair follicle in the outer ear canal.

Causes include trauma (from cotton buds, etc.), increased humidity (e.g., wearing hearing aid), and swimming in dirty water, etc. Diabetics and patients with skin conditions – eczema and psoriasis – are at a higher risk of developing otitis externa.

> Infective: bacterial – localised (furuncle) or diffuse
> Fungal: *Aspergillus niger*, *Candida* species
> Viral: herpes zoster/simplex
> Reactive: eczema, seborrheic dermatitis, psoriasis

Principles of Management

Otitis externa is a very painful condition. Adequate oral analgesia, suction clearance of the discharge, and topical steroid/antibiotic eardrops are the treatments. If the ear canal is narrow, insert a pope wick (Otowick) which by its hygroscopic nature absorbs the moisture in the ear canal and swells up. It relieves pain by splinting effect and by reducing the edema.

Acute (Suppurative) Otitis Media (AOM/ASOM)

Acute inflammation of part or whole of the mucosa of middle ear cleft (Tympanic cavity, Eustachian tube and Mastoid air cell system).

Common pathogens – *S. pneumoniae*, *H. influenzae*, *Branhamella catarrhalis*, *Staphylococcus* species. Organisms enter via Eustachian tube usually following a bacterial URTI. Highest incidence is in 2–7-year-olds, but any age may be affected.

Patients classically present with pain, pyrexia, deafness, and discharge. Patients with pain from Eustachian tube dysfunction or glue ears are often misdiagnosed to have ASOM.

The course of AOM follows the stages below:

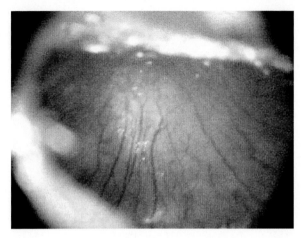

FIGURE 5.7 A photo-otoscopic view of the right ear showing acute otitis media. Note the injected and prominent vessels on the tympanic membrane

Stage of Hyperemia

In the early stage of AOM, ear discomfort and mild earache are common. In most instances, disease may resolve completely without further progression.

On examination, the ear drum appears congested and inflamed.

Treatment: reassurance, analgesics, and observation. Use of antibiotics is controversial (Fig. 5.7).

Stage of Suppuration

Patient presents with severe earache, fever, and malaise. Exudates forms in the middle ear as a result of infection. The ear drum appears inflamed and bulging (Fig. 5.8).

Treatment: analgesics/antipyretics

Oral antibiotics (Gram-positive bacteria)

Amoxicillin/Co-Amoxiclav or
Erythromycin or cephalexin

Decongestant nose drops: xylometazoline/ephedrine

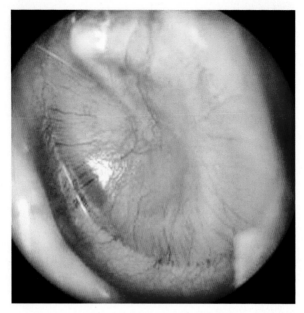

FIGURE 5.8 An advanced case of acute otitis media. Note the bulging left tympanic membrane and the displacement of the handle of the malleus into a more horizontal position and consequent alteration of the light reflex

Stage of Perforation

Increased middle ear pressure causes a spontaneous pinhole perforation of the tympanic membrane and lets the mucopurulent discharge out. This causes instant relief of pain and ear discomfort (Fig. 5.9).

Treatment: oral antibiotics less effective
Topical antibiotic ear drops: chloramphenicol, ciprofloxacin, Sofradex or Genticin.

Stage of Coalescence

Following tympanic perforation, the AOM may either

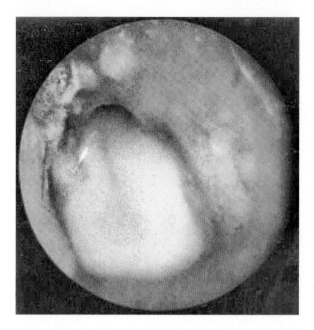

FIGURE 5.9 Rupture of an ischemic area of the tympanic membrane with the release of "pus" and relief of symptoms

(a) Resolve completely with closure of eardrum perforation or
(b) Cause prolonged otorrhoea due to persistent eardrum perforation or
(c) Result in temporary (usually) middle ear effusion (glue ear)

Complications of AOM: Facial Nerve Palsy, Acute Mastoiditis, Chronic Otitis Media, Vestibular Disturbances, Sensorineural Hearing Loss

Acute Mastoiditis

Spread of infection to mastoid air cells can cause abscess formation leading to swelling and redness behind the pinna. The pinna looks prominent as it is pushed forward and outward.

Treatment: admission and broad spectrum IV antibiotics. I&D of abscess ± mastoid exploration is required in most cases. Early treatment of acute mastoiditis prevents intracranial spread of infection.

Key Points

Real ENT emergencies are few. Prompt diagnosis, early and precise intervention is essential for the conditions mentioned below:

> Potential airway problems – angioedema, floor of mouth infections, acute epiglottis
>
> FB in throat/esophagus
>
> The time to do a tracheostomy is when you think of it.
>
> Epistaxis is the loss of blood and may require emergent fluid replacement and cross matching and should not be trivialized
>
> Orbital cellulitis – can cause permanent blindness in the affected eye in a matter of hours
>
> Septal hematoma
>
> Acute mastoiditis
>
> Urgent removal if FB in nose/ears happens to be a battery

Chapter 6
Urological Emergencies

Heman E.S. Prasad, Shafiq Ahmed, Rohan J. Mammen, Mathew Thomas, and Kim Mammen

Clinical Case Scenario 1: Paraphimosis

Case Presentation

A 72-year-old male, who had been catheterized 24 h ago for retention of urine, presented with pain and swelling on the tip of his penis. On examination, the catheter was in position draining clear urine, but the glans penis was found to be exposed, and his prepuce was swollen and edematous. He was

H.E.S. Prasad, M.B.B.S., M.S. (Surgery) (✉) • S. Ahmed,
M.B.B.S., M.S., DNB (Urology)
Department of Urology, Christian Medical College and Hospital,
Ludhiana, Punjab, India
e-mail: hemanprasad@gmail.com

R.J. Mammen, M.B.B.S. • K. Mammen, M.S., MCh, DNB, FRCS, FACS
Department of Urology, Christian Medical College and Hospital,
Ludhiana, Punjab, India

M. Thomas, M.B.B.S., MRCS
Department of Urology, Royal Liverpool and Broadgreen University
Hospitals, Liverpool, UK

I. Shergill et al. (eds.), *Surgical Emergencies in Clinical Practice*,   99
DOI 10.1007/978-1-4471-2876-2_6,
© Springer-Verlag London 2013

unable to pull the foreskin back over the glans penis. A tight band was noted proximal to the swollen prepuce.

Features of History and Examination

Paraphimosis is the entrapment of a retracted foreskin behind the coronal sulcus. It is often iatrogenic and can be prevented by returning the prepuce to cover the glans following penile manipulation for procedures like catheterization, endoscopic procedures, or during cleaning. Paraphimosis most commonly occurs after urethral catheter placement, but in the younger population, there may be a history of preceding sexual activity, such as masturbation. Preexisting phimosis is thought to be a risk factor.

The foreskin becomes trapped behind the corona over a period of time, typically due to a tight, constricting band of tissue. This constricting band impairs blood and lymphatic drainage from the distal glans and prepuce, causing it to engorge and become edematous. Paraphimosis should be treated promptly since the constricted band may result in vascular compromise, gangrene, necrosis, and potentially auto-amputation.

On examination, the foreskin is retracted and forms a constricting band, which causes edematous swelling of the distal part of the glans. The penis has to be carefully examined for the extent of the edema. The color of the glans and palpation of the glans provides information on the viability of the glans. A normal glans is soft and pink, whereas a tense and bluish-colored glans can point to vascular compromise.

Management

Paraphimosis should be treated promptly as it is a very painful condition and timely action prevents tissue loss. Treatment of paraphimosis is reducing the foreskin. This involves manually compressing the glans and prepuce with steady pressure, to decrease the edema, and gently moving the foreskin back to its normal position, perhaps with the aid of a lubricant, cold compression, and local anesthesia as necessary. It is useful at this point to administer adequate analgesic cover prior to attempting any manipulation since paraphimosis is a painful condition – this can be done by dorsal penile nerve or penile ring block.

Other rarely used techniques can also be used, with the aim of reducing the edema, allowing effective manual retraction of the foreskin over the glans.

An "iced glove" can be used where after applying topical anesthetic gel to the glans and prepuce, the area is immersed in ice water. This may reduce the swelling.

The "Dundee technique" starts with a ring block using local anesthesia. Then a small gauge needle (25G) is used to make multiple punctures into the edematous foreskin. This allows the drainage of edematous fluid. This procedure should be covered with broad-spectrum antibiotics.

Gauze pieces soaked in 50% dextrose can be wrapped around the glans and prepuce. It can reduce the edema by osmosis. Hyaluronidase has been described to help reduce the paraphimosis. It is injected into the edematous prepuce. Degradation of hyaluronic acid by hyaluronidase enhances diffusion of trapped fluid between the tissue planes to decrease the preputial swelling.

The traditional surgical management is the dorsal slit, whereby the constricting ring is cut. Two hemostats are applied to crush the foreskin at the 12 o'clock position perpendicular to the corona. The prepuce between the hemostats is cut, and this releases the constricting band. At a later stage, a formal circumcision will have to be carried out to prevent recurrences of paraphimosis. Patients with evidence of significant glans penis ischemia, with necrosis and sloughing of the foreskin and/or glans, will require operative debridement of the devitalized tissue.

Key Learning Points

- Paraphimosis, if left untreated, can lead to gangrene of the penis and tissue loss (auto-amputation).

- Manual reduction – with constant circumferential pressure on the glans and prepuce – is the most effective technique for successful reduction.
- Other techniques are used to reduce edema prior to manual reduction, and include concentrated sugar applications, hyaluronidase injections, and multiple punctures all of which aid in decreasing the edema and swelling.
- Circumcision has to be done at a later date to prevent a recurrence.
- Prevention and early intervention are key elements in the management of paraphimosis.

Clinical Case Scenario 2: Penile Fracture

Case Presentation

A 27-year-old male presented to A&E with pain, swelling, and discoloration of his penis. He initially gave conflicting descriptions of how this had occurred, but then confessed that he had been celebrating earlier that evening, and when he returned he engaged in vigorous intercourse with his partner. While she was on top, straddling him, he heard a snap and he lost his erection. He felt a sharp pain and at the same time he lost his erection. The patient was able to pass urine without any problems. Examination of the penis revealed a purplish discoloration of the shaft of the penis resembling an eggplant. Deviation of the shaft to one side was noted. Palpation of the shaft revealed a step deformity.

History and Examination

Penile fracture is an injury caused by the rupture of the tunica albuginea, surrounding the corpus cavernosum of the penis. The tunica albuginea has high tensile strength requiring a pressure in excess of 1,500 mmHg to achieve rupture. Most common cause is enthusiastic sex, especially with the woman-on-top position. Other etiologies include events such as falls and penile manipulation. Certain practices like "Taqaandan," (Kurdish for "to click") make penile fractures more common. Taqaandan is the forceful bending of the distal erect penis while stabilizing the proximal penile shaft, until a click is heard. Treatment of penile fracture is surgical.

History of hearing a "snap" or a "popping" sound followed by immediate detumescence and minimal to severe sharp pain, depending on the severity of injury, points to a possible penile fracture. There could also be history of a direct blow or forced bending of the tumescent penis. There could be difficulty in voiding, and if there is associated urethral injury, blood may be noticed at the external meatus. Often, the patient gives history of a sexual act prior to the injury wherein his penis slipped out, hitting the perineum or the pubis of his female partner.

On examination, the normal appearance of the penis is distorted due to penile deformity, swelling, and ecchymosis (known as "eggplant" deformity). Soft tissue swelling of the penile skin, penile ecchymosis, and hematoma formation are apparent. Penile hematoma is confined to the penile shaft if the Buck's fascia is intact or may form a "butterfly-pattern" hematoma over the perineum, scrotum, and lower abdominal wall if Buck's fascia has ruptured. Sometimes in a cooperative patient, a blood clot may be palpable at the site of fracture and the clot may be felt as a discreet firm mass over which the penile skin may be rolled (known as the "Rolling sign"). There could be urinary retention that mostly is secondary to urethral injury or periurethral hematoma that causes bladder outlet obstruction.

Principles of Acute Management

A penile fracture is a very painful condition and adequate analgesics should be given in the emergency room. The mainstay treatment is surgical intervention to restore the penis back to the preinjury state, preserve penile length, and allow normal voiding.

Even in the presence of clinically evident penile fracture, it must be remembered that the incidence of associated urethral injury ranges from 2% to 10%. If a urine microscopic examination reveals blood along with clinically evident urethral injury, a retrograde urethrography will help rule out urethral injury. Alternatively, careful urethroscopy can also be attempted to assess the integrity of the urethra before exploring the fracture site. In uncertain cases of penile fracture, diagnostic cavernosography or MRI of the penis may be helpful.

Surgery consists of exploration of the wound and repair of the tunica after evacuation of the hematoma. A circumcising degloving incision is best suited for wound exploration. Delayed absorbable suture like polydiaxanone may be used for tunica repair. Methylene blue injection into the corpora cavernosum can be used intraoperatively to exact the location of the rent in the tunica; this reduces the operative time and also unnecessary dissection.

An artificial saline-induced erection may be induced to test for watertight integrity of the repair before closing. Patients are advised to abstain from sexual activity for 7–10 weeks after surgical repair. Partial and complete urethral transections that are clean with adequate length of urethra amicable to repair are repaired with a primary anastomosis over an indwelling catheter. A urinary diversion via a suprapubic cystostomy can be done for wound healing to complete. Drains usually are not placed. Complications of penile fracture are erectile dysfunction (due to a cavernosospongiosal fistula), abnormal penile curvature, painful erections, and formation of fibrotic plaques.

Key Learning Points

- Penile fracture is rupture of the corpus cavernosum due to blunt trauma to the erect penis.
- Most common cause is enthusiastic sexual activity with the woman-on-top position.
- Treatment is mainly surgical with exploration and repair of the torn tunica albuginea.

- Urethral injury occurs in 2–10% of cases.
- Complications can range from penile curvature, erectile dysfunction high-flow priapism, and fistulae.

Clinical Case Scenario 3: Priapism

Case Presentation

A 52-year-old male presented to accident and emergency department with a painful erection lasting around 6 h. A month ago, he had given a history of erectile dysfunction and was reviewed by his GP. He had tried PDE5 inhibitors with little success and had been prescribed intracorporeal alprostadil. He had been shown how to use it, and this was his second attempt at using it. On examination, an erect tender penis was noted though the glans was not firm.

History and Examination

Priapism derives its name from the Greek God of fertility, Priapus. It is a pathological state of penile erection and is defined as persistent penile erection for more than 4 h that continues beyond or is unrelated to sexual stimulation. The pathophysiology of priapism is mainly the failure of detumescence and can be due to the under-regulation of arterial inflow (known as high-flow or arterial priapism) or, more commonly, the failure of venous outflow (known as low-flow or veno-occlusive priapism). Stuttering or intermittent priapism is recurring episodes of priapism interspersed with detumescence.

Priapism is classified into three types; non-ischemic (high-flow) priapism, ischemic (low-flow) priapism, and recurrent or stuttering priapism. The condition is most common between the ages of 5–10 years and 20–50 years. Timely treatment is very important in management of priapism to prevent any permanent long-term complications like erectile dysfunction (see Fig. 6.1).

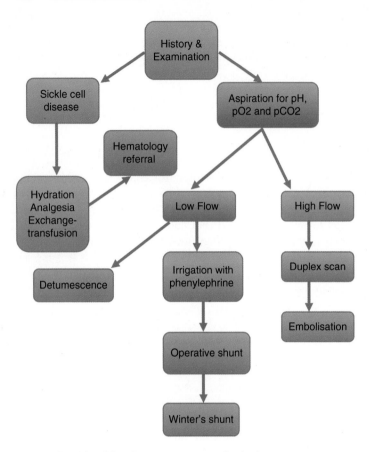

FIGURE 6.1 Algorithm for management of priapism

The corpus cavernosum is engorged in priapism where as the corpus spongiosum is spared and not engorged. Use of prescribed drugs like antihypertensives, anticoagulants, antidepressants, and other psychoactive drugs, or recreational drugs such as alcohol, marijuana, or cocaine, can predispose to priapism. The combination of intracavernosal agents and other drugs is the cause of priapism in approximately 21–80% of the adult Western population. Previous episodes of priapism should be elicited. Past medical history including sickle cell disease, leukemia, or advanced malignancies should be elicited. History of trauma, neurological conditions, or infections (malaria, rabies, scorpion sting) should be ruled out.

Blood gas testing and color duplex ultrasonography are currently the most reliable diagnostic methods of distinguishing ischemic from nonischemic priapism. Blood aspirated from the corpus cavernosum with ischemic priapism is hypoxic and therefore dark, while blood from the corpus cavernosum with nonischemic priapism is normally oxygenated and therefore bright red. A blood gas analysis will give exacting determinants. Blood from ischemic priapism will mostly have a pO_2 of less than 30 mmHg, a pCO_2 of more than 60 mmHg, and a pH <7.25.

Management

The goal of the management of all patients with priapism is to achieve detumescence and preserve erectile function. The principle of treatment of priapism is to reduce the intracavernosal pressure to restore venous drainage for penile detumescence and establish adequate arterial perfusion of cavernosum-corpus, to decrease the hypoxic state of cavernosum-corpus, and finally to prevent structural damage and fibrosis. A penile nerve block with a long-acting local anesthetic such as bupivacaine without epinephrine increases patient comfort and improves patient cooperation. Initial treatment of priapism in an emergency setting consists of phenylephrine intracavernous injection therapy and aspiration using 19G butterfly needle. A mixture of a 1ml ampoule of phenylephrine (1 mL: 1,000 µg) diluted with 9 mL of normal saline is used. Using a 29-gauge needle, 0.3–0.5 mL of the preparation is injected into the corpora cavernosa, waiting 10–15 min between injections. This is followed by aspiration of the corpora cavernosa and then saline irrigations. Blood pressure and pulse rate must be measured during administration of phenylephrine. This is repeated, if necessary, over several hours. Phenylephrine is less effective in priapism of more than 48-h duration because ischemia and acidosis impair the intracavernous smooth muscle response to sympathomimetics. Management of sickle cell disease–associated priapism will include oxygenation, analgesics like intravenous morphine, hydration, alkalization, and exchange transfusions to increase the hematocrit value to greater than 30% and to decrease the hemoglobin-S value to less than 30%. These treatments should not delay progression to intracavernous treatment.

If such a therapy fails, or if there is prolonged ischemic priapism, shunt procedures are recommended. The objective of a shunt is to allow blood to drain from the corpora cavernosa, bypassing the veno-occlusive mechanism of these structures. Several different shunts are described. A cavernoglanular shunt (made with a scalpel is known as the Ebbehoj technique, and when made using a large core biopsy needle is known as the Winter technique) is probably the easiest to perform and associated with least complications. The Al-Ghorab shunt procedure is a more aggressive open surgical cavernosal shunt where a small piece of the tunica albuginea is excised. The Quackels or Sacher shunt causes proximal shunting of blood and is done by creation of a window between the cavernosum-corpus and corpus spongiosum. The Grayhack shunt is a proximal cavernosal-saphenous shunt that surgically connects the proximal corpora cavernosum to the saphenous vein. All these shunts mainly attempt to reverse the priapism state by shunting blood out of the rigid corpora cavernosa into low-pressure areas.

The initial management of nonischemic priapism should be observation. Selective arterial embolization is recommended for the management of nonischemic priapism.

Key Learning Points

- Priapism is defined as persistent penile erection for more than 4 h that continues beyond or is unrelated to sexual stimulation.
- Priapism is to be initially attempted to be treated with saline/phenylephrine irrigation.

- Distal shunts (e.g., Winter's) and proximal shunts (e.g., Quackel's) work on the principle of draining blood from the priapic tumescent penis.
- Al-Ghorab shunt involves an iatrogenic rent in the tunica albuginea.
- Nonischemic priapism has to be observed for spontaneous detumescence.

Clinical Case Scenario 4: Acute Urinary Retention

Case Presentation

A 69-year-old male patient presented with inability to pass urine for more than 12 h. He was having symptoms of urgency, frequency, feelings of incomplete emptying during micturition, and nocturia over the last few months. During the last 12 h, he found it more and more difficult to pass urine till he was unable to pass urine at all. There was no history of trauma. On examination, there was a palpable tender mass in the suprapubic region. A rectal examination showed a benign feeling moderately enlarged prostate. The rectum was otherwise empty and no masses were felt.

History and Examination

Acute urinary retention (AUR) refers to the sudden inability to pass urine. Various events can precipitate AUR, including medication, infection, general anesthesia, and performance of various diagnostic genitourinary procedures. Almost all patients with acute urinary retention will have an identifiable predisposing factor.

Factors precipitating acute urinary retention include:

- Benign enlargement of prostate
- Malignant enlargement of prostate
- Medications – for example, anticholinergics, α-adrenergic agonists, or antihistamines

- Genitourinary instrumentation
- Postoperative retention – due to anesthesia, pain, perioperative fluids, immobilization
- Neurological – radical pelvic surgery (damage to pelvic
  parasympathetic plexus) and spinal cord injury or cauda
  equina syndrome

On examination, a palpable bladder is usually felt in the
suprapubic region (this can be difficult in obese patients). This
is associated with dullness to percussion and a desire to void
during palpation. A rectal examination is mandatory to assess
the size and consistency of the prostate, as well as to assess the
rectum and anal tone. The external genitalia have to be examined for phimosis or meatal stenosis. In cases of urethral
trauma, the perineal region has to be specifically examined
for any hematoma due to a urethral injury. All women require
a pelvic examination, careful neurological assessment, and an
ultrasound scan of the pelvis as minimum investigation.

Management

Acute urinary retention is usually treated by catheterization.
This can be urethral or suprapubic depending on circumstances and is usually done in accident and emergency
departments on admission. This initial treatment relieves the
immediate distress of a full bladder and prevents permanent
bladder damage. The residual volume must be recorded and
a urinanalysis is carried out. If it is not possible to pass a
urethral catheter or if urethral catheterization is contraindicated (suspected urethral injury) then a suprapubic catheter
should be inserted. Strict instructions should be given to
monitor urine output in those patients with high post catheterization residuals (usually >1 L), as they are more prone to
diuresis and may need intravenous fluid replacement (if
hourly urine output >200 mL/h for 2 or more consecutive
hours).

Bloods must be taken for assessment of renal function and
full blood count.

If the patient is dehydrated, prompt rehydration and reas-
sessment is pertinent. Catheter drainage should then be

maintained until the etiology of the obstruction is treated appropriately.

Precipitated retention usually does not recur once the precipitating cause is removed. 50% of those with spontaneous retention will experience a second episode within 1 week and 70% within 1 year. Recurrence is 90% for men with an initial peak urinary flow rate less than 5 mL/s.

To prevent recurrence of AUR in men, an α-blocker is prescribed 48 h prior to TWOC (Trial of voiding Without Catheter). If the TWOC is successful, this needs to be continued lifelong. For those with large prostates (volumes >40 g), it is reasonable to add a 5-α-reductase inhibitor (the effects of these will not be seen for several months). Side effects such as postural hypotension and retrograde ejaculation (α-blocker) and loss of libido or impotence (5-α-reductase inhibitor) need to be discussed with patient prior to starting therapy. A word of warning for patients with deranged renal function with retention (obstructive uropathy): they should not be started on medical therapy and should proceed to surgical treatment or long-term catherization.

For those who fail medical management, surgical treatment is the next option. The most common procedure is the transurethral resection of prostate.

For those who fail medical management and are unfit or reluctant for surgery, clean intermittent catheterization or long-term catheterization are viable options.

Key Learning Points

- Acute urinary retention almost always has an underlying cause, most common in elderly men being benign prostatic hyperplasia.
- Emergency treatment involves catheterization or suprapubic urinary diversion.
- Decision for further definitive treatment is done after a trial of voiding without catheter.
- Uroselective α-Blocker can be prescribed for preventing recurrences.
- Those with obstructive uropathy should not have a TWOC and proceed to surgical management.

Clinical Case Scenario 5:
Renal (Ureteric) Colic

Case Presentation

A 42-year-old male presented with sudden onset pain in the left loin radiating to the groin with no pain on the right side and no previous history of any urological problem. He described the pain as sudden, sharp, and gripping in nature. There were no aggravating or relieving factors. Simple analgesia did not help. The pain was associated with nausea and vomiting and he could not be in a comfortable position. On examination, there was some tenderness in the left renal angle. Urine dipstick showed microscopic hematuria.

History and Examination

The classic presentation of renal colic is excruciating unilateral flank or lower abdominal pain of sudden onset that is not related to any precipitating event and is not relieved by postural changes or simple analgesia.

It usually radiates from the loin to groin, prompting the patient to seek medical attention. Striking without warning, the pain is often described as being worse than childbirth, broken bones, gunshot wounds, burns, or surgery. There may be marked tenderness in the costovertebral angle and/or the right or left lower quadrant of the abdomen. There may be hematuria, either macroscopic or microscopic. As the stone progresses down the ureter, the pain tends to migrate caudally and medially. The referred pain is due to common innervations of the upper ureter and the testis (T11-T12) and the lower ureter and the inner side of the upper part of the thigh (L1, through genitofemoral nerve). The pain of renal colic may be associated with nausea, vomiting, and frequent or urgent urges to urinate, which may be painful. Blood in the urine (hematuria) occurs frequently with kidney stones. This blood may be visible or microscopic. Occasionally, abdominal aortic aneurysm pain may mimic renal colic. It is two to three times more common in males than in females. In women, ovarian torsion and ectopic pregnancy can be mistaken for renal/ureteric colic. In men, epididymitis or even testicular torsion may mimic the symptoms of distal ureteral stones. On examination, there could be renal angle / flank tenderness during an episode of colic.

Management

The severity of the pain of a ureteric colic is such that it often prompts one to seek care at a hospital emergency room. The management of ureteral calculi begins with a focused history that includes duration and evolution of symptoms. The physical examination is often more valuable for ruling out non-urologic disease. Pain relief can be obtained with oral painkillers (e.g., NSAIDs), but usually it requires stronger analgesics such as intravenous opiates. The diagnosis is often made based on clinical symptoms alone, although confirmatory tests are usually performed.

Plain-film radiography of the kidneys, ureters, and bladder (KUB) is usually the first investigation at admission. Stones that contain calcium, such as calcium oxalate and calcium phosphate stones are mostly detected by plain film radiography. The size and location of these calculi can be documented. Plain-film radiography has its inherent drawbacks such as the calculi being obscured by stool or bowel gas, or the bony pelvis or transverse processes of vertebrae. Sulfur-containing stones are relatively radiolucent (eg., cystine stones), while pure uric acid stones are completely radiolucent.

Renal ultrasound works best in the setting of relatively large stones within the renal pelvis or kidney and sometimes at the PUJ.

The intravenous pyelogram (IVP) provides useful information about the stone (size, location, radio density) and its environment (calyceal anatomy, degree of obstruction), as well as the contralateral renal unit (function, anomalies, etc.). Compared with abdominal ultrasonography and KUB radiography, intravenous pyelography has greater sensitivity

(64–87%) and specificity (92–94%) for the detection of renal calculi. The renal function must be kept in mind while performing an IVP, especially in those who are predisposed to renal failure. Contrast-induced nephropathy is one of the leading causes of hospital-acquired acute renal failure.

Noncontrast CT scan as an initial assessment of renal colic is a fast and accurate imaging modality. It readily identifies all stone types, except indinavir stones (formed in people taking antiretroviral in the treatment of HIV) in all locations. Its sensitivity (95–100%) and specificity (94–96%) is adequate to use it as a diagnostic tool. CT is now becoming the primary modality for investigating renal colic.

Microscopic examination of the urine is a critical part of the evaluation of a patient thought to have renal colic. Gross or microscopic hematuria is only present in approximately 85% of cases. The lack of microscopic hematuria does not eliminate renal colic as a potential diagnosis.

Initial treatment consists of analgesia to control the pain. This is best achieved using a NSAID (e.g., diclofenac). If this is not enough, then opiate analgesic is used. Once this has been achieved, the next step is to formulate a strategy for managing the stone. Stones less than 4 mm usually pass spontaneously (90–98%). α-blockers assist in stone passage. However, if a stone <4 mm has not passed within 4 weeks, it needs intervention and removal.

Indications for immediate stone removal are:

- Pain which fails to respond to analgesia
- Impaired renal function
- Prolonged obstruction (>6 weeks)

If the patient is septic, immediate management consists of drainage of the obstructing kidney (JJ stent or nephrostomy) and treatment of sepsis with antibiotics. The stone can be dealt with once the sepsis is settled.

Treatment options for stones depend on size and position.

- Proximal stones <1 cm ESWL or ureteroscopy
- Proximal stones >1 cm ESWL, ureteroscopy or PCNL (after pushing the stone into kidney)
- Distal stones ESWL or ureteroscopy

Key Learning Points

- Acute renal colic is a painful emergency which makes the patient promptly seek a doctor.
- Diagnosis can be made from history and classical loin-to-groin-pain.
- Noncontrast helical CT scan is the standard imaging modality for ureteral stone localization.
- NSAIDs analgesics are the choice for pain relief.
- Stone less than 4 mm usually pass out spontaneously; larger stones need definitive intervention.

Clinical Case Scenario 6: Testicular Torsion

Case Presentation

A 15-year-old male presented with sudden onset of right testicular pain for 6 h. Pain developed when he was walking home from school. This was present only on the right side of the scrotum. Simple analgesia took the edge off the pain but did not relieve it completely. There was no history of trauma or UTI or similar pain in the past. The intensity of the pain was increasing. On examination, the patient was in severe pain with difficulty in moving. He had a tender right testis, and examination was difficult due to the pain. Elevation of the testis did not reduce the pain. The testes were high riding and more horizontal than normal.

History and Examination

Testicular torsion is an absolute urological emergency that must be differentiated from other complaints of testicular pain since any delay in diagnosis and management can lead to loss of the testicle. There is twisting of the spermatic cord, which in turn cuts off the blood supply to the testicle. Incidence of torsion in males younger than 25 years is approximately 1 in 4,000.

All prepubertal and young adult males with acute scrotal pain should be considered to have testicular torsion until proven otherwise. Torsion more often involves the left testicle. Among the cases of testicular torsion that occur in the neonatal population, 70% occur prenatally and 30% occur postnatally.

The commonest symptom is sudden onset of severe unilateral scrotal pain. Torsion is also noted to occur with activity, can be related to trauma in 4–8% of cases, or can develop during sleep. This condition is most common between ages 7 and 12. It can be confused with torsion of the appendix of the testis, or epididymitis in children. Some patients have a history of recurrent scrotal pain that has resolved spontaneously. This history is suggestive of intermittent torsion of the testicle. On physical examination, the involved testicle is typically very tender and patient has exquisite pain. There may be ipsilateral loss of the cremasteric reflex in patients with testicular torsion. To differentiate from acute epididymitis, upon elevation of scrotum usually there is no relief of pain (elevation may improve the pain in epididymitis, known as Prehn's sign). There is no role of investigation in diagnosis of torsion, if torsion is suspected, surgical exploration is warranted. The differential diagnosis of the acutely painful scrotum includes testicular torsion, trauma, epididymitis/orchitis, incarcerated hernia, varicocele, idiopathic scrotal edema, and torsion of the appendix testis. Sometimes the appendix of the testis, a vestigial structure of membranes attached to some testes, may also undergo painful twisting. In most males, the testes are attached posteriorly to the inner lining of the scrotum by the mesorchium. When the mesorchium terminates early and does not attach the testis, this is called a bell clapper deformity, and this is a predisposing factor for testicular torsion in non-neonates.

Management

Adequate analgesic pain relief should be administered as testicular torsion is typically very painful. Usually intravenous opiates are required. Antiemetics are given to prevent vomiting. Clinically it can be difficult to differentiate torsion from other diagnosis, and if there is any doubt of the diagnosis, a scrotal exploration is indicated. Irreversible ischemic injury to the testicular parenchyma may begin as soon as 6 h after occlusion of the cord, and as time progresses, the chance of viability of the testis decreases. After 24 h, the chance of viability of the testis is almost 0%.

A midline scrotal incision is used for scrotal exploration. On exploration, if the testicle is not viable, it must be removed (orhchidectomy). The anatomic abnormality that predisposed the testicle to torsion may be bilateral; therefore, exploration and fixation of the contralateral testis is recommended. If testicular torsion is diagnosed early, a near 100% salvage rate is possible. Orchiopexy, even though reduces the chances of torsion in future, does not guarantee against future torsion.

Complications of testicular torsion may include infarction of testicle, loss of testicle, infection, infertility secondary to loss of testicle, and cosmetic deformity.

Key Learning Points

- Torsion is a true urological emergency and time should not be wasted in investigations if clinical diagnosis is suggestive of torsion testis.
- It is more common in the pediatric age group.
- Prophylactic orchiopexy of the unaffected testicle is performed.
- Torsion testis is most commonly misdiagnosed as acute epididymo-orchitis.

Further Reading

Shergill I, Arya M, Patel H, Gill IS. Urological Emergencies in Hospital Medicine. London: Markallen Group; 2007.

Chapter 7
Maxillofacial Emergencies

Tahwinder Upile, Waseem Jerjes, Colin Hopper, N. Patel, and Janavikulam Thiruchelvam

Introduction

It is only recently that maxillofacial surgery ceased to be just a dental specialty and now requires formal surgical/medical training for specialist registration. It remains, however, founded

T. Upile, B.Sc. (hons), M.Sc., M.S., M.D., FRCS (Gen Surg), FRCS (OTO), FRCS (ORL-HNS), DFFP, FHEA, MRCGP (✉)
Department of ENT, Barnet and Chase Farm Hospital, Enfield, Greater London, UK

Head and Neck Unit, University College London Hospitals, London, UK
e-mail: mrtupile@yahoo.com

W. Jerjes, B.Sc. (hons), Ph.D., M.Sc., BDS, MBBS
Department of ENT, Barnet and Chase Farm Hospital, Enfield, Greater London, UK

C. Hopper, FRCS, M.D.
Head and Neck Unit, University College London Hospitals, London, UK

N. Patel, FRCS
Head and Neck Unit, Department of ENT, Southampton University Hospitals, Southampton, UK

J. Thiruchelvam, FRCS, M.D.
Oral Maxillofacial Unit, Head and Neck Department, Barnet and Chase Farm Hospitals, Greater London, UK

I. Shergill et al. (eds.), *Surgical Emergencies in Clinical Practice*, 119
DOI 10.1007/978-1-4471-2876-2_7,
© Springer-Verlag London 2013

in dentistry requiring many of the skills and attributes learned in general dental or oral surgical practice. Medical specialists as a part of emergency treatment and patient management may be called upon to treat dental injuries and maxillofacial trauma. Once again, ATLS management protocols must be adhered to with early airways management (bearing in mind a potential cervical spine injury) from any significant injury. The multidisciplinary role of emergency surgical airways management may include emergency, general, ENT, and maxillofacial surgeons. The place of several transtracheal catheters (grey/brown venflon) connected to oxygen to buy time until a definitive airway must not be forgotten.

Many undergraduate curricula do not include maxillofacial surgery teaching and now reserve OMF for postgraduate students; this leaves the junior surgeon poorly prepared for initial clinical duties. It is essential that multidisciplinary care is entered into early, and that when required, appropriate referral is made at the opportune time to more senior and/or specialist teams. We have selected the cases based upon their frequency of presentation, need for correct initial management, and due to the medicolegal consequences of poor management. Other more complex surgical emergencies may be found in specialty-specific texts.

Clinical Case Scenario 1: Dentoalveolar Injuries

Case Presentation

A 16-year-old male comes to A&E with history of injury in school with avulsion of upper anterior tooth. He was bullying one of the junior pupils, who punched him in the face. There was no loss of consciousness, and the teacher brought him to hospital immediately. He has no past history of medical problems and is not on any medication.

Key Features in History and Examination

History

General questions pertaining to any other trauma victims (loss of consciousness, other injuries, immediate treatment, etc.). Specific questions pertaining to avulsed teeth – time since avulsion, where was the tooth found, how was it brought to A&E (dry, milk, water, saline).

Examination

Make sure the tooth is intact. Exclude other head and neck injuries and fractures. Check cheek sensation.

Principles of Acute Management

Initially ATLS protocol, then concentrate on management specific to maxillofacial surgery. Clean the tooth with saline. Hold the tooth with the crown. Do not scrub the root surface, just clean it with saline. If indicated, X-rays may be taken. Earliest implantation and stabilization of the tooth into its socket is essential.

Discussion

Dental injuries are common and are frequently associated with other facial trauma. The spectrum of dental injury is varied (including Crown fracture, crown root fracture, root fracture, periodontal ligament concussion, subluxation, luxation). Injury to the crown can range from chipping of enamel to exposure of pulp. This can be very painful and is best treated by a dentist. Remember to look for tooth fragments in the adjacent lacerations, confirmed by X-rays (Fig. 7.1). Prescribe analgesic and advice to see a dentist

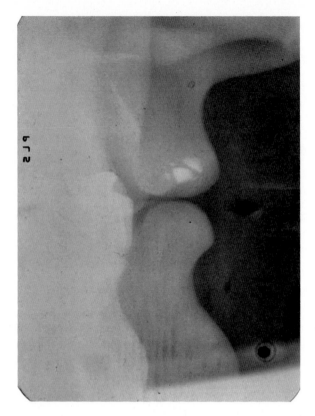

FIGURE 7.1 X-ray demonstrating tooth fragments adjacent to laceration

ASAP. Retain all large pieces because they can be bonded back onto the tooth.

Various levels of the root can also be fractured. This should be suspected when the tooth is loose and should be confirmed with an X-ray. If the root tip is fractured, the tooth should be splinted and advice given to contact a dentist. Prescribe analgesics and antibiotics.

Luxated (partially displaced) tooth (Fig. 7.2) should be reduced and splinted. X-rays should be taken to rule out fracture of the root. Advice patients to contact dentist ASAP.

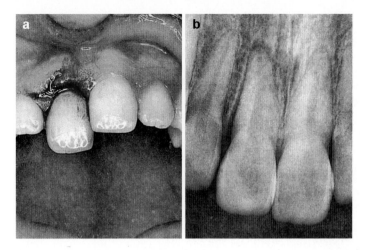

FIGURE 7.2 Luxated tooth and X-ray excluded fracture of the root

Avulsed teeth (out of the socket) needs rapid treatment. Tooth is best stored in cold milk or patients own mouth until it is reimplanted. Wash with cold running saline and hold it with the crown.

If a whole dentoalveolar segment is fractured, the whole segment has to be reduced and splinted. Any associated gingival tear should be sutured. Impressions can be taken to guide the reduction of teeth and also useful to make a custom-made splint.

Clinical Case Scenario 2: Dental Infection

Case Presentation

A 14-year-old patient presents with a 6-day history of swelling in his left cheek. It was preceded by toothache and is now progressively getting worse. On arrival, he is apyrexial and otherwise well, but looks flushed. He was unable to attend for

PE lesson today and his mother took him to the dentist, who immediately referred him to the on call ENT team.

Key Features in History and Examination

History

Ask for duration, source of infection, tooth pain, difficulty in breathing, or swallowing. Ask about diabetes and immunodepression. Previous dental history and imaging taken.

Examination

Assess the extent of the swelling (determine which dental space is involved). Look out for the source of infection (skin, teeth, etc.). Grave signs include trismus, raised floor of mouth, unable to swallow, and drooling of saliva.

Principles of Acute Management

If airway is potentially compromised, one needs urgent airway management. Inform anesthetist for assessment. Try to avoid a tracheostomy. Steroids can be given to reduce edema.

Appropriate antibiotics should be given immediately (to cover cocci and anaerobes). Necessary radiographs (Fig. 7.3) should be taken to identify the source. Drainage is indicated if there is collection of pus. At the same time, the source of infection should be dealt with (e.g. extraction).

Blood tests should be done to rule out undiagnosed diabetes or other hematological conditions (leukemia).

Discussion

Acute facial swelling due to dental infection can be life threatening. It can progress rapidly in some cases. Therefore, urgent management is critical. In early stages, oral antibiotics are enough with urgent attention to the source of infection.

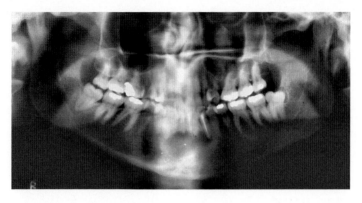

FIGURE 7.3 Orthopantomogram (*OPG*) showing source of infection

In severe cases, urgent admission for IV antibiotics is important. Continuous monitoring of progress or airway compromise is necessary till the time of definitive management. If there is pus collection, drainage at the earliest is necessary with removal of the source of infection. Depending on the teeth, various spaces can be involved. These include:

1. Canine space
2. Buccal space
3. Submandibular space
4. Submental space
5. Sublingual space
6. Submasseteric space
7. Pterygomandibular space
8. Parapharyngeal space
9. Temporal space

Ludwigs Angina

Ludwig's angina is an acute and potentially life-threatening cellulitis involving, sublingual, submental, and submandibular spaces often due to dental infection. The tongue is swollen, floor of mouth is raised, and the patient will have difficulty in swallowing (Fig. 7.4). This will lead to airway obstruction if not intervened early. This condition therefore needs immediate management of airway and drainage of the above spaces.

FIGURE 7.4 Image of patient with Ludwig's angina

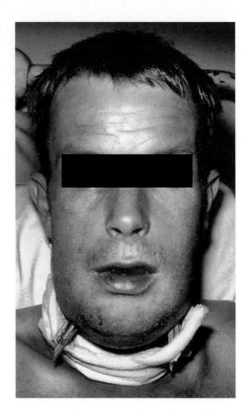

Admission to ITU may be necessary. General principles of dental infection management as above apply, but urgent attention to airway and drainage is critical.

Clinical Case Scenario 3: Mandibular Fractures

Case Presentation

A 25-year-old male comes to *accident and emergency department* with pain and difficulty in closing the mouth after a fight in a nightclub. He was punched once after he insulted his friend's

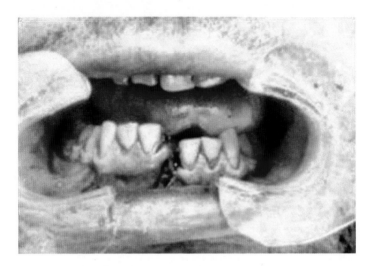

FIGURE 7.5 Step deformity in a patient with mandibular fracture

partner. There was no loss of consciousness and he remembers the incident vividly.

Key Features of History and Examination

Acute examination according to ATLS principles. A head injury of some form is to be expected and should be managed appropriately.

History

After initial assessment, essential history to be obtained are nature of injury, altered occlusion, numbness of lip and tongue, loss of teeth, and location of pain. Also, presence of previous skeletal deformity and temporomandibular joint problems should be determined.

Examination

Once other injuries are ruled out, look out for deformity, site of swelling, and tenderness; document the teeth present or missing, presence of loose teeth, step deformity (Fig. 7.5),

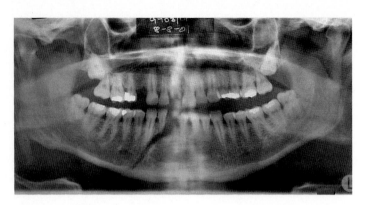

FIGURE 7.6 Orthopantomogram showing mandibular fractures

altered occlusion, sublingual hematoma, numbness of lower lip and tongue, reduced mouth opening, and mobility of fracture site if other findings are not convincing.

Principles of Acute Management

After initial management of ATLS is through and once a clinical diagnosis of a fractured mandible is made, confirmation is required with radiographs. Two X-rays are required orthopantomogram (Fig. 7.6) and PA mandible (Fig. 7.7).

In some cases, CT may be required. Start the patient on antibiotics and give adequate pain killers. If the fracture site is grossly displaced, reduction and temporary splinting with wires around the teeth will reduce the pain and bleeding.

Discussion

Mandibular fracture is one of the common bony maxillofacial injuries. The common cause is interpersonal violence. The other causes include road traffic accidents, sports injuries, fall, and industrial accidents. All these patients should be examined

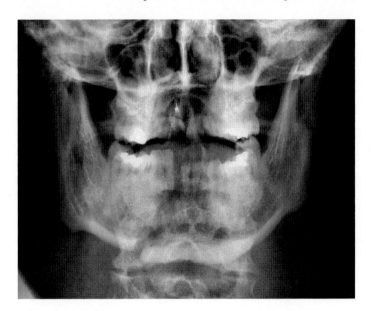

FIGURE 7.7 PA mandible X-ray

for other bony and dental injuries. The common sites of mandibular fracture are shown in Fig. 7.8.

This includes condyle, coronoid, ramus, angle, body, parasymphysis, and symphysis. Commonly, the mandible will fracture in two places. Therefore, if one fracture is identified, always look carefully at other sites. Due to the presence of teeth, most mandibular fractures are compound fractures and have a potential to get infected. Therefore, antibiotics should be prescribed.

There are several methods of fixation of the fracture. This includes closed reduction and fixation (intermaxillary fixation) and open reduction and internal fixation (ORIF) with plates. With the advent of mini-plates and screws, ORIF has been widely accepted as the treatment of choice. In general condyle, ramus and coronoid are treated with closed reduction and fixation. Angle, body, symphysis and parasymphysis are treated with ORIF with mini-plates. Two plates are required

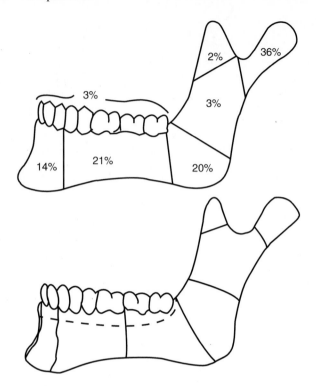

FIGURE 7.8 Common sites of mandibular fracture

in front of the mental foramen and one plate behind it (AO principle). Usually the fracture is approached intraorally. In selected cases, extraoral approach is indicated.

Clinical Case Scenario 4: Soft Tissue Injuries

Case Presentation

A 30-year-old male comes with a laceration to his left cheek (Fig. 7.9). He denies any knowledge of how he received the injury but is accompanied by a group of friends, with various injuries to their face and limbs.

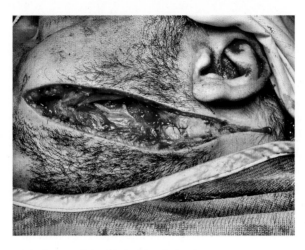

FIGURE 7.9   Laceration of left side of cheek

Key Features of History and Examination

Acute examination according to ATLS principle.

History

After initial assessment, essential histories to be obtained are circumstances of the incident, offending weapon, other lacerations, and amount of blood lost. Other injuries must be excluded!

Examination

Examination should include the depth of the lacerations and involvement of vital structures, that is, facial nerve and parotid duct. Tissue loss, if any, should also be identified. The wounds should be photo-documented for later reference so dressing is not disturbed. Swabs, etc., should be taken before further wound contamination.

Principles of Acute Management

Initially, according to ATLS principles, and then specific to laceration, control of bleeding is essential prior to thorough examination to identify the structures involved.

Antibiotic and tetanus cover should be given. Thorough debridement of the wound is essential. The vital structures such as nerves, parotid duct should be repaired prior to suturing the tissue in layers.

Discussion

Soft tissue injuries can be classified into contusion, abrasion, laceration, avulsion, burns (chemical, thermal). Circumstances of the injury are essential as they will give insight into the associated injuries and contamination.

All particulate matters and foreign bodies in the wound should be removed or they will result in traumatic tattooing. Petroleum-based liquids such as grease and oil should be removed by solvents like acetone or ether. Type of laceration will give an idea of the nature of injury. Sharp objects produce a clean straight cut. Stellate laceration is usually due to blunt injuries.

Most lacerations to the head and neck are simple one, caused by a fall. These wounds are cleaned and closed primarily. Some lacerations are large and can be associated with tissue loss or damage to vital structures. In the neck, any laceration deep to the platysma should be evaluated with care to identify damage to other vital structures. Stab wounds should be examined with care as the depth is unpredictable with a small entry wound.

Bite Wounds

Bite wounds (Fig. 7.10) are associated with high infective risk. This is not only due to the presence of highly infective bacterial flora in the mouth (animals and human beings) but also due to the multiple types of injury. The animal bites usually

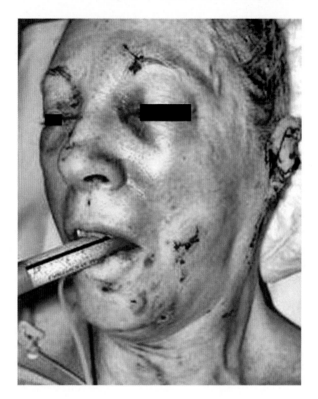

FIGURE 7.10 Bite on face and cheek with infection

are penetrating type with a small entry wound. The infective flora is lodged deep into the tissue as the entry point would seal quickly with clots. Animal bites, especially of dogs, are polymicrobial. It includes *Staphylococcus aureus*, β-hemolytic *Streptococcus*, anaerobic Bacteroides and Fusobacterium and *Pasteurella multocida* (especially in cat bites). Human bites have a higher concentration of Bacteroides but also contain *Staphylococcus* and α-hemolytic *Streptococcus*.

Principles of Treatment of Bite Wounds

As head and neck are highly vascularized, the bite wounds can be closed primarily. However, the wound should be irrigated copiously and debrided appropriately. Especially the small punctured wound should be opened and irrigated well to its depth. Broad-spectrum antibiotics should be prescribed in addition to tetanus cover.

Clinical Case Scenario 5: Post–Dental Extraction Bleeding

Case Presentation

A 55-year-old patient comes to *accident and emergency department* with H/O bleeding from the mouth. He had a tooth extracted by his dentist in the morning. It has not stopped since, and he gives a history, only after prompting, of shaving injuries taking an extremely long time to stop bleeding.

Key Features in History and Examination

History

Has it been continuous/profuse? History of bleeding disorders, hypertension. Medications the patient is on (anticoagulants, aspirin, clopidogrel, etc.).

Examination

Examine to make sure the patient is hemodynamically stable. Measure blood pressure/pulse. Under a good light, examine the socket after suctioning. Look at the status of the extraction socket and look out for the source of bleeding (from gingival/extraction socket). Is there an obvious bleeding vessel?

Principles of Acute Management

Consider emergency circulatory management scenario. Measure pulse, BP, and control the local hemorrhage with local pressure (biting on a moist/adrenaline-soaked gauze). If the patient has been bleeding a lot, it may be necessary to start an IV line to take bloods for FBC, coagulation screen, group and save or cross-match blood, and to give fluids. If it continues to bleed, look at the source. Give local anesthetic. The extraction socket needs to be compressed. If the gingiva is bleeding, it may need to be sutured. If the bleeding is from the socket, it needs to be packed with surgical and the socket sutured. Tranexamic acid mouthwash or systemic tranexamic acid (oral/IV) can be given. An X-ray needs to be done if there is a suspicion of retained roots or foreign body in the socket. Check for systemic cause if all the above measures fail and treat it accordingly.

Discussion

Post-extraction bleeding is not uncommon. Most of the patients stop with local measures.
   Local causes include

1. Gingival tear
2. Gingiva not closely adapted to bone
3. Failure to have compressed the extraction socket
4. From the socket due to retained roots or raw bony socket

The systemic causes include

1. Hypertension
2. Bleeding/coagulation disorders

Key Points

1. ATLS management protocols must be adhered to with early airways management (bearing in mind a potential cervical spine injury) from any significant injury.
2. The multidisciplinary role of emergency surgical airways management may include emergency, general, ENT, and maxillofacial surgeons.
3. Mandibular fracture is one of the common bony maxillofacial injuries. The common cause is interpersonal violence. The

other causes include road traffic accidents, sports injuries, fall, and industrial accidents. All these patients should be examined for other bony and dental injuries. The common sites of mandibular fracture are shown in Fig. 7.8.

Acute facial swelling due to dental infection can be life threatening.

Bite wounds (Fig. 7.10) are associated with high infective risk. This is not only due to the presence of highly infective bacterial flora in the mouth (animals and human beings) but also due to multiple types of injury.

Chapter 8
Cardiothoracic Surgical Emergencies

Narain Moorjani and Stephen Westaby

Introduction

Cardiothoracic surgery is a highly subspecialized field of surgery and a specialty where morbidity and mortality rates have been directly correlated with multidisciplinary team-working, level of surgical expertise and the presence of state-of-the-art facilities, in the diagnosis, treatment and management of complications. Importantly, cardiothoracic surgery evokes an emotion of high surgical standards, grace and prestige in the public eye, as well as among other healthcare professional.

Interestingly, very few surgical trainees will have an opportunity to rotate through cardiothoracic surgery. This chapter has been written with those junior doctors in mind, as well as providing a refresher for juniors already in cardiothoracic surgery or those who may have passed through it during their rotations. Within this subspecialty, junior trainees are very unlikely to actually perform the surgery, although they may be allowed to do parts of procedures, such as vein grafting in coronary artery bypass grafting, depending on their level of

N. Moorjani, MBChB, MRCS, M.D., FRCS (C-Th) (✉)
Department of Cardiothoracic Surgery, Papworth Hospital,
University of Cambridge, Cambridge, UK
e-mail: narain.moorjani@doctors.org.uk

S. Westaby, B.Sc., FRCS, M.S., Ph.D., FESC, FACC, FECTS, FICA
Department of Cardiothoracic Surgery, John Radcliffe Hospital,
Oxford, UK

I. Shergill et al. (eds.), *Surgical Emergencies in Clinical Practice*, 137
DOI 10.1007/978-1-4471-2876-2_8,
© Springer-Verlag London 2013

clinical experience. Thus, the emphasis of this chapter has been on highlighting the five commonest cardiothoracic emergencies that they may come across, either in a specialized unit or indeed, more commonly, while in a typical district general hospital, where cardiothoracic facilities may not exist. One of the underlying messages has been to learn how to diagnose the emergencies expeditiously and be in a position to be able to communicate the findings to the subspecialized cardiothoracic center for urgent and immediate transfer. Importantly, surgical treatment, as opposed to medical therapy, in a cardiothoracic center will be the only method of securing a safe and satisfactory outcome for many of these patients.

Clinical Case Scenario 1: Aortic Dissection

Case Presentation

A 68-year-old gentleman presents to the accident and emergency department with sudden onset, tearing chest pain radiating into the back, associated with dyspnea. His past medical history includes a long-standing history of hypertension, which was being treated pharmacologically. On examination, he is tachycardic with a pulse of 110 bpm and hypertensive with a blood pressure of 160/95, equal in both arms. Auscultation reveals an early diastolic murmur. All peripheral pulses are present.

Key Features of History and Examination

- Aortic dissection occurs following a tear in the intima of the aortic wall, which allows ingress of blood into the media and splitting of the aortic wall between the internal and external elastic media. Clinical features depend on the extent of the dissection and organ involvement.
- Acute aortic dissection usually presents with sudden onset of pain, typically tearing in nature. The site of the

pain may help to indicate the location of the disease process, with chest pain suggestive of ascending aortic involvement and back pain indicating descending aortic involvement. The majority of dissections originate in the ascending aorta (65%), followed by the descending aorta and aortic arch.

- The sudden onset chest pain of ascending aortic dissection needs to be differentiated from other causes of acute chest pain including myocardial infarction and pulmonary embolus.
- The patient may be hypotensive if tamponade is present, or hypertensive, if the autoregulatory processes are disturbed following stripping of the baroreceptors by the dissection process.
- Other clinical features include an early diastolic murmur (suggestive of aortic regurgitation), unequal blood pressure in the upper limbs and absent peripheral pulses.
- Complications of aortic dissection depend on the extent of the disease process and may include:

    (a) Aortic rupture and cardiac tamponade
    (b) Acute aortic regurgitation and subsequent volume-overload-induced heart failure
    (c) Organ (cardiac, cerebral, visceral or limb) malperfusion and subsequent ischemia

Principles of Acute Management

Investigations for acute aortic dissection include:

Electrocardiogram (ECG)

This may show signs of left ventricular hypertrophy (secondary to long-standing hypertension) or acute myocardial ischemia (secondary to dissection of the coronary ostia). Remember, occasionally the ECG may also be normal!

Chest Radiograph (CXR)

This may demonstrate a widened mediastinum.

Echocardiography

Although transthoracic images may show evidence of aortic dissection, transesophageal echocardiography (TOE) is able to more clearly delineate the dissection flap in the ascending aorta. Passing the TOE probe may, however, precipitate hypertension and further disruption of the intimal tear. There is also a blind spot in the distal ascending aorta and proximal aortic arch during TOE.

Computed Tomography (CT)

This is usually the diagnostic investigation of choice, as it can image the entire aorta and its main branches (brachiocephalic, carotid, subclavian, mesenteric, renal and femoral arteries), demonstrating the extent of the dissection and allowing determination of the surgical strategy. In patients with renal impairment, there may be a risk of contrast-induced nephropathy.

Magnetic Resonance Imaging (MRI)

This is usually able to provide excellent quality diagnostic images but is not always readily available.

Aortography

Historically, it was the gold standard imaging for the diagnosis of aortic dissection but is less commonly used due to risk of precipitating aortic rupture.

The principles of managing patients with acute aortic dissection include:

1. Blood pressure control using a combined alpha- and beta-adrenergic antagonist (e.g., labetalol) to reduce the aortic

shear stress. In addition, nitrates and nitroprusside may also be required. In patients with hypotension, the diagnosis of cardiac tamponade or myocardial ischemia (secondary to aortic dissection) should be considered. They should be resuscitated with volume and inotropes and undergo immediate surgery.

2. Emergency surgery for patients with acute dissection involving the ascending aorta (Stanford type A or DeBakey type I or II). The principles of surgery are to resect the entry point of the dissection (intimal tear) and restore antegrade flow through the true lumen, thereby preventing the catastrophic complications of acute ascending aortic dissection, which include rupture and tamponade; severe aortic regurgitation and heart failure; and organ (coronary and cerebral) malperfusion and ischemia.

3. Conservative management for patients with dissection not involving the ascending aorta (Stanford type B or DeBakey type III), with blood pressure control and serial aortic imaging. Surgery should only be undertaken in this group of patients if there are signs of rupture or impending rupture; signs of extension or unremitting pain; or evidence of visceral (renal or mesenteric) or limb ischemia. Endovascular stent grafting is being increasingly used for the management of descending thoracic aortic dissection.

Discussion

Acute dissection of the ascending aorta is a cardiothoracic surgical emergency, where the diagnosis needs to be established early and the presenting symptoms need to be distinguished from other causes of acute chest pain. Surgery is mandated in patients with acute aortic dissection involving the ascending aorta. Without surgery, 1–2% of these patients die per hour within the first 24–48 h, and only 25% survive at 2 weeks, as a result of rupture, tamponade, severe aortic regurgitation, myocardial ischemia, stroke or organ malperfusion. In patients where the ascending aorta is not involved, conservative management is advocated, as the surgery does not improve short- or long-term outcomes and is associated with an increased risk of paraplegia. Surgery is only indicated in these patients if there is evidence of rupture, dissection extension or organ ischemia. In the long term, all patients with acute aortic dissection require strict blood pressure control to protect the residual native thoracic aorta. One of the main predictors of long-term survival is patency of the false lumen within the residual native aortic arch and descending aorta. Serial aortic imaging is necessary to identify aneurysmal expansion of this residual native aorta and determine if subsequent aortic surgery is required.

Key Points

1. Acute aortic dissection is relatively rare, with an incidence of 30–35 per million. It occurs more commonly in men and in patients over the age of 60. Recognized risk factors include hypertension, connective tissue diseases (e.g., Marfan syndrome), bicuspid aortic valve, atherosclerosis, and pregnancy.
2. Acute ascending aortic dissection usually presents with sudden onset of chest pain, typically tearing in nature, but needs to be differentiated from myocardial infarction and pulmonary embolism.
3. Contrast-enhanced CT thorax provides excellent images of the entire aorta and its branches to determine the management strategy.
4. Emergency surgery is required for acute dissection involving the ascending aorta, whereas patients with dissection only involving the descending aorta are usually managed conservatively.
5. In the long term, blood pressure control and serial thoracic aortic imaging is required.

Clinical Case Scenario 2: post-infarct Ventricular Septal Rupture

Case Presentation

A 67-year-old gentleman presents with new onset left-sided chest pain. Three days previously, he had sustained an anterior myocardial infarction for which he was thrombolysed. Associated with this, he is dyspneic at rest. On examination, he is tachycardic with a pulse of 116 bpm and hypotensive with a blood pressure of 95/55. Auscultation reveals a harsh pansystolic murmur loudest over the left sternal edge in the 5th intercostal space and inspiratory crackles over both lungs bases.

Key Features of History and Examination

- Acute complications of myocardial infarction include ventricular septal rupture (VSR), papillary muscle rupture and left ventricular rupture. These diagnoses need to be considered in a patient who acutely hemodynamically deteriorates 2–6 days following a transmural myocardial infarction.
- Ventricular septal rupture and papillary muscle rupture should be considered in patients presenting with a new systolic murmur following myocardial infarction. The murmur with post-infarct VSR is often associated with a palpable thrill over the left sternal edge. The pansystolic murmur associated with papillary muscle rupture and subsequent mitral regurgitation is usually more prominent over the apex.
- The development of pulmonary edema and heart failure following post-infarct VSR is determined by the site and size of the infarction and the magnitude of the left to right shunt across the defect.
- Ventricular septal rupture is usually associated with a transmural myocardial infarction, secondary to complete

occlusion of the left anterior descending artery (70%), resulting in an anterior post-infarct VSR, or posterior descending artery (30%), resulting in an inferior post-infarct VSR.

Principles of Acute Management

Investigations for post-infarct ventricular septal rupture include:

Electrocardiogram (ECG)

This may demonstrate right axis deviation, right bundle branch block or complete heart block, as well as signs of recent anterior or inferior myocardial infarction.

Chest Radiograph (CXR)

This usually shows increased pulmonary venous congestion and pulmonary edema.

Echocardiography

This is used for the definitive diagnosis of post-infarct VSR and allows differentiation from post-infarct papillary muscle rupture. The site and magnitude of the left to right shunt is also delineated, using color flow Doppler, as well as the left and right ventricular function, which are important prognostically.

Coronary Angiography

This is used to demonstrate the coronary lesions to determine the need for coronary artery bypass grafting during surgery. Simultaneous ventriculography can also demonstrate the shunt but is rarely used due to the risk of contrast nephropathy in these patients.

Right Heart Catheterisation

This can provide measurement of oxygen saturations, with a "step-up" (>9%) from the right atrium to the pulmonary artery, associated with oxygenated blood shunting from left to right across the defect. The pulmonary-to-systemic flow ratios (Qp:Qs) can then be used to calculate the shunt ratio, which roughly correlates with size of the defect.

Once diagnosed, these patients are hemodynamically optimized without delaying surgery by administering diuretics and an inotropic agent that also vasodilates, such as dobutamine and also by inserting an intra-aortic balloon pump (IABP). This reduces the systemic vascular resistance and the left to right shunt, thereby augmenting the cardiac output, coronary artery blood flow and organ perfusion.

Definitive management of patients with post-infarct ventricular septal rupture involves emergency surgical repair, with concomitant coronary artery bypass grafting, as indicated by the coronary angiogram. In patients with cardiogenic shock and multiorgan failure, it may be prudent to treat them conservatively initially, as emergency surgery carries a very high mortality in this cohort of patients. Following median sternotomy, surgery is usually performed via an incision through the infarcted left ventricular anterior or inferior wall, with the aid of cardiopulmonary bypass support. A bovine pericardial patch is then sutured to healthy endocardium deep in the left ventricle to exclude the infarcted septum and septal defect from the high-pressure area of the left ventricle. More recently, percutaneous closure of post-infarct ventricular septal rupture has been performed with varying results.

For patients who present with contained post-infarct LV rupture, the infarct exclusion technique (described above for post-infarct VSR) is employed. Acute non-contained LV rupture is invariably fatal. Patients with post-infarct papillary muscle rupture require either reimplantation of the papillary muscle (for partial rupture) or mitral valve replacement (for complete rupture).

Discussion

Post-infarct ventricular septal rupture is a cardiac surgical emergency. The incidence of post-infarct VSR is 1–2% of all myocardial infarctions but has fallen considerably with improved thrombolysis and primary angioplasty. Acute hemo-dynamic management involves reducing the systemic vascular resistance to decrease the left to right shunt and thereby improve organ perfusion. This is achieved by using an intra-aortic balloon pump, diuretics and inodilators. Definitive man-agement is by surgical repair of the defect using an infarct exclusion technique. More recently, percutaneous closure has been introduced into the clinical arena but with varying out-comes. In patients with post-infarct VSR treated medically, only 20% survive 1 month and 5% survive at 1 year. In com-parison, the operative mortality for patients with post-infarct VSR is 30–40%. In hospital survivors following surgery, the 5-year survival is 75% with a New York Heart Association (NYHA) symptom status I-II in 80% of these patients.

Between 10% and 25% of patients develop residual or recurrent shunts following surgical repair of post-infarct VSR. The majority of these, especially if small (Qp:Qs < 2) and asymptomatic, can be treated conservatively with diuretic therapy. Spontaneous closure may occur; otherwise percuta-neous or operative intervention is required. Patients with chronic post-infarct VSR can be treated either surgically with direct patch closure, attached to the thickened, fibrotic, scarred edges of the VSR, or percutaneously.

Key Points

1. Post-infarct VSR occurs following a transmural myocar-dial infarction and usually involves the left anterior descending artery (70%), resulting in an anterior VSR.
2. Patients usually present with new onset chest pain, acute hemodynamic instability and a harsh pansystolic murmur, 2–6 days following an acute myocardial infarction.

3. Definitive diagnosis is made by echocardiography, although right heart catheterization or pulmonary artery catheter measurements can demonstrate a "step-up" in oxygen saturations from the right atrium to the pulmonary artery.
4. Patients with post-infarct VSR should be hemodynamically optimized using inodilators, diuretics and placement of an intra-aortic balloon pump.
5. Definitive management involves surgical repair using an infarct exclusion technique.

Clinical Case Scenario 3: Cardiac Trauma

Case Presentation

Following a stabbing to the left side of his chest, a 23-year-old gentleman presents to the accident and emergency department with acute dyspnea and chest pain. On examination, he is tachycardic with a pulse of 118 bpm and hypotensive with a blood pressure of 80/60. Inspection reveals markedly distended neck veins and a 5 cm linear stab wound in the 4th intercostal space at the left sternal edge. On auscultation, muffled heart sounds are heard, as well as reduced breath sounds over the left lung.

Key Features of History and Examination

- Cardiac tamponade should be suspected in all patients who present with penetrating cardiac trauma. The clinical diagnosis of tamponade can be made with the aid of Beck's triad, which includes hypotension, distended neck veins and distant or muffled heart sounds.
- Other specific signs that may be present with cardiac tamponade include:

  (a) Pulsus paradoxus, which is defined as an abnormally excessive fall in the systolic blood pressure on inspiration

>10 mmHg. Normally on inspiration, there is a slight fall in the systolic blood pressure (<5 mmHg).

(b) Kussmaul's sign, which is defined as a rise in the jugular venous pressure during spontaneous inspiration. Normally, the jugular venous pulse decreases with the negative intrathoracic pressure associated with inspiration. This sign may, however, not be present until any coexistent hypovolemia is corrected with fluid resuscitation.

- During examination of these patients following penetrating cardiac trauma, it is important to identify any associated injuries, such as a left hemopneumothorax.
- Although cardiac tamponade may initially have a protective effect by reducing the volume of the blood loss, it will eventually compromise cardiac diastolic filling, as the pericardial sac acts as a fixed volume box.
- Following penetrating cardiac trauma, only a small volume (100–200 ml) of fluid is required to compromise cardiac filling, as opposed to the larger volumes (up to 2 l) required with chronic pericardial effusions associated with malignancy, as the pericardium does not distend significantly in the acute phase.
- The anatomical position of the heart in relation to the anterior chest wall determines the frequency with which each chamber is involved in penetrating cardiac trauma, with the right ventricle being the most anterior chamber: right ventricle (45%), left ventricle (35%), right atrium (15%) and left atrium (5%).

Principles of Acute Management

Most victims of massive penetrating cardiac trauma die at the scene. For those reaching the hospital, management of patients with penetrating cardiac or mediastinal trauma must follow Advanced Trauma Life Support (ATLS) guidelines, identifying associated injuries related to the airway, breathing and circulation. Inserting two large bore intravenous cannulae allows for rapid fluid resuscitation, as required. Although certain investigations help to confirm cardiac tamponade, it should be diagnosed clinically and treated immediately to decompress the heart.

Investigations for penetrating cardiac trauma include:

Electrocardiogram (ECG)

This may demonstrate low-voltage QRS complexes or electric alternans, secondary to a pericardial collection, caused by the heart moving within a fluid-filled sac. ST elevation may also be present.

Chest Radiograph (CXR)

This may show pneumopericardium or globular enlargement of the heart caused by the pericardial collection. This, however, is not present in all cases as the pericardium may not have had time to stretch. The CXR may also show any associated injuries, such as hemopneumothorax.

Echocardiography

This is used for definitive diagnosis of cardiac tamponade, demonstrates a significant pericardial collection with the heart swinging freely within the pericardial sac and diastolic collapse of the right ventricle and atrium. Associated injuries such as septal defects and valvular lesions also need to be identified on echocardiography.

Although paraxiphoid pericardiocentesis can help to improve the patient's clinical condition by decompressing the heart, the definitive treatment of cardiac tamponade secondary to penetrating cardiac trauma is open drainage of the pericardial collection and surgical repair of the cardiac injury.

According to the ATLS guidelines, emergency resuscitative thoracotomy should be used for patients following penetrating trauma (not blunt trauma) within 10 min of the onset of pulseless electrical activity (PEA). It is performed through a left anterolateral thoracotomy in the 4th intercostal space. Through this access, the therapeutic options include evacuation of the pericardium, open cardiac massage, repair of any cardiac injuries or clamping of the descending aorta (to stop distal bleeding and increase coronary and cerebral perfusion). If greater exposure to the heart is required, the left anterior thoracotomy can be extended across the sternum as a bilateral "clam shell" incision. This allows access to the great vessels and both sides of the heart but both internal thoracic arteries need to be ligated. If the patient is relatively stable and appropriate equipment is available, a median sternotomy is often preferred.

Once access to the heart and great vessels has been obtained, the main priority is to achieve hemostasis and repair of the cardiac injury. Either direct pressure or a Foley catheter to occlude the hole is used until direct repair is feasible. For posterior cardiac wounds, the heart may need to be lifted out of the pericardial sac but it is important to avoid inducing air embolism during this procedure. In these and other circumstances, cardiopulmonary bypass support may be required. Although uncommon (<5%), damage to the coronary arteries by the penetrating injury may require bypass grafting.

Discussion

The diagnosis of cardiac tamponade needs to be suspected in all patients who present with penetrating cardiac trauma. The diagnosis should be made clinically in patients with Beck's triad, which includes hypotension, distended neck veins and muffled heart sounds. Echocardiography, when performed, demonstrates a significant pericardial collection with diastolic collapse of the right ventricle and atrium. Although pericardiocentesis can temporarily improve the hemodynamic status of the patient, definitive management involves open drainage of the pericardial tamponade and surgical repair of the cardiac wound. Emergency room thoracotomy should only be used in patients following penetrating cardiac trauma and within 10 min of the onset of pulseless electric activity.

Key Points

1. Following penetrating cardiac trauma, prompt diagnosis of cardiac tamponade is essential by clinical signs including Beck's triad. Pulsus paradoxus and Kussmaul's sign may also be present.
2. Although cardiac tamponade may initially have a protective effect by reducing the volume of the blood loss, it will eventually compromise cardiac diastolic filling.
3. These patients may benefit from prompt decompression by paraxiphoid pericardiocentesis but definitive management requires operative closure of penetrating cardiac wound.
4. Emergency room thoracotomy should only be used in patient following penetrating cardiac trauma and within 10 min of the onset of pulseless electric activity.
5. If stable, median sternotomy gives better access to the pericardium and great vessels if time permits.

Clinical Case Scenario 4: Infective Endocarditis

Case Presentation

A 68-year-old lady presents with increasing dyspnea over the past few weeks associated with recurrent fever, rigors and night sweats. She is known to have mitral valve prolapse and has recently undergone a dental extraction, without any antibiotic cover. On examination, she is pyrexial with a temperature of 38.1°C, tachycardic with a pulse of 106 bpm but is normotensive with a blood pressure of 125/75. On auscultation, she has a pansystolic murmur, heard loudest at the apex, radiating to the axilla and inspiratory crackles heard over both lung bases.

Key Features of History and Examination

- Infective endocarditis has an incidence of 2–4 cases per 100,000 persons per year with native valves and 0.5–1% per year following valve replacement surgery.
- Patients with underlying valvular pathology or septal defects are susceptible to infective endocarditis, as these lesions produce non-laminar flow, thereby inducing platelet-fibrin thrombus formation. Subsequent bacterial colonization from an interventional procedure (such as dental extraction, colonoscopy or surgery) results in vegetation formation and potential embolization or spread into the surrounding tissues.
- Infective endocarditis usually affects the left-sided valves, with involvement of the mitral valve more common than the aortic valve. Only 5% of cases involve the tricuspid valve, with the pulmonary valve rarely being affected.
- Although fever is the commonest symptom, infective endocarditis can present in a number of ways, including:

    (a) Clinical features of infection, such as fever, night sweats, rigors, weight loss and malaise.
    (b) Clinical features of immune complex deposition, such as Roth spots (retinal boat-shaped hemorrhage with a pale center), splinter hemorrhages (thin reddish-brown lines in the nail bed), Osler's nodes (painful pulp infarcts on fingers, toes, palms or soles), Janeway lesions (painless flat palmar or plantar erythema) or arthralgia.
    (c) Clinical features of the cardiac lesion, such as a new or changing murmur; heart block or heart failure.
    (d) Clinical features of emboli (including cerebral, splenic, renal or lower limb) resulting in organ infarct or abscess formation.

Principles of Acute Management

In patients with suspected infective endocarditis, the key principles in managing these patients include:

(a) Establishing the diagnosis (using clinical presentation, blood cultures and echocardiography).
(b) Commencing broad-spectrum antibiotics (once the blood cultures have been taken).
(c) Surveillance with serial blood tests (inflammatory markers and blood cultures) and echocardiography to determine whether the patient requires surgical intervention.

The diagnosis of infective endocarditis can be made with the aid of Duke's criteria (Table 8.1) by establishing two major criteria; one major and three minor criteria; five minor criteria; or pathological evidence of active infective endocarditis (from the surgical specimen or postmortem).

Streptococcus or *Streptococcus* (45%), *Staphylococcus* or *Staphylococcus* (35%) and *Enterococcus faecalis* (10%) are the commonest organisms causing native or late (>2 months)

TABLE 8.1 Duke's criteria

Major criteria
Three positive blood cultures (taken 12 h apart) showing typical organisms, such as *Streptococcus viridans*, *Staphylococcus aureus*, or *Enterococci*
Evidence of endocardial infection, such as demonstration of a vegetation, abscess, prosthetic valve dehiscence or new regurgitation on echocardiography
Minor criteria
Predisposing factors (such as intravenous drug abuser, underlying valvular lesion or septal defect)
Fever >38°C
Embolic or vascular phenomena (such as splinter hemorrhages or vasculitis)
Immunological phenomena (such as Osler's nodes or Roth spots)
Serology consistent with infective endocarditis
Blood cultures compatible with, but not typical for, endocarditis
Echocardiographic findings consistent with infective endocarditis and not covered by major criteria

prosthetic valve endocarditis. *S. aureus* and *S. epidermidis* (50%), Gram-negative bacilli and fungi are the commonest organisms causing early (<2 months) prosthetic valve endocarditis. If the organism is unknown, broad-spectrum antibiotics are prescribed using benzylpenicillin and gentamicin (which covers *Streptococcus*) or vancomycin and gentamicin (if *Staphylococcus* is suspected). Once the blood cultures results are available, appropriate antibiotic therapy can then be prescribed, tailored to the causative organism.

The majority of patients presenting with infective endocarditis are managed medically without the need for operative intervention. Surgery is usually reserved for patients with heart failure; infective endocarditis caused by highly resistant or virulent organisms, such as fungi or *S. aureus*; local invasion (producing heart block, periannular abscesses, fistula or leaflet perforation); prosthetic valve dehiscence; recurrent emboli despite appropriate antibiotic therapy; or the presence of vegetations >10 mm.

Discussion

The main principles of surgery for patients with infective endocarditis include debridement of infected tissues, closure of cardiac defects and valve repair or replacement. In patients with aortic valve endocarditis extending into an aortic root abscess, reconstruction with a bovine pericardial patch may be possible; otherwise aortic root replacement with an aortic homograft is required. In patients with mitral and tricuspid valve endocarditis, valve repair is the preferred option, especially if <50% of the valve is affected. In intravenous drug abuser patients with tricuspid valve endocarditis, it may be necessary to excise the valve leaflets without valve replacement in order to reduce the risk of recurrence but this can only be done in the absence of any significant pulmonary hypertension. Operative mortality is approximately 5–10% for patients with native valve endocarditis and 10–20% for patients with prosthetic valve endocarditis.

Similarly, 5-year survival is better for patients with native valve endocarditis (80%) compared to those with prosthetic valve endocarditis (60%).

Key Points

1. Infective endocarditis has an incidence of 2–4 cases per 100,000 persons per year with native valves and 0.5–1% per year following valve replacement surgery.
2. Patients with infective endocarditis can present with clinical features of the cardiac lesion, infection, immune complex deposition or systemic embolization.
3. Echocardiography is the mainstay in the diagnosis of infective endocarditis, allowing identification of any vegetation present and the spread of infection into the surrounding structures.
4. Surgery for infective endocarditis should be performed for patients with heart failure, highly resistant organisms, local invasion (producing heart block, periannular abscesses, fistula or leaflet perforation), prosthetic valve dehiscence, recurrent emboli or vegetations >10 mm.
5. The main principles of surgery for patients with infective endocarditis include debridement of infected tissues, closure of cardiac defects and valve repair or replacement.

Clinical Case Scenario 5: Aortic Transection

Case Scenario

A 28-year-old gentleman is brought to the accident and emergency department following a high-speed head-on collision in a road traffic accident. He presents with severe interscapular pain, as well as marked right thigh and pelvic pain. On examination, he is tachycardic with a pulse of 115 bpm, hypotensive with a blood pressure of 90/55 and hypoxic with oxygen saturations of 91%. Although present, both left and right lower limb pulses were weaker than those of the upper limbs.

Key Features of History and Examination

- The diagnosis of aortic transection should be considered in all patients that have experienced sudden deceleration injury, such as following a road traffic accident or a high fall.
- The patient may not present with any symptoms or signs directly related to the aortic injury but transection should be suspected in all patients with severe blunt thoracic trauma, especially in those with upper rib (1st–3rd), sternal and scapula fractures. Associated injuries may also be present, including:

  (a) Intrathoracic injuries, such as pulmonary contusion (resulting in hypoxia), tracheobronchial disruption, myocardial contusion and esophageal disruption
  (b) Extrathoracic injuries, such as pelvic and femoral fractures and abdominal visceral injury

- Stretching or dissection of the aortic adventitia may cause retrosternal or interscapular pain. Furthermore, compression of the surrounding structures by a periaortic hematoma may result in dysphagia, stridor, dyspnea or hoarseness.
- Hemodynamic compromise secondary to hypovolemia results in tachycardia, hypotension and oliguria.
- Transection of the aorta usually occurs at the aortic isthmus between the origin of the left subclavian artery and the ligamentum arteriosum. The deceleration injury causes the greatest strain at the junction of mobile structures (such as the aortic arch) and relatively immobile structures (such as the descending aorta, which is fixed in place by the intercostal arteries, ligamentum arteriosum and surrounding structures).
- Complete transection of the thoracic aorta is usually fatal, with 85% of patients with aortic transection dying at the scene. For those who reach the hospital alive, only the media and intimal layers of the aorta are involved. The adventitia and surrounding mediastinal tissues remain intact, containing

the rupture and thereby maintaining aortic luminal continuity. Pulses distal to the aortic disruption may, however, be weaker than those proximal to the lesion.

Principles of Acute Management

Investigations for traumatic aortic rupture include:

Chest Radiograph (CXR)

As part of the initial trauma screening, a widened mediastinum on CXR may be suggestive of aortic transection. Most trauma CXRs, however, are taken in an anteroposterior (AP) projection and this artificially enlarges the mediastinal silhouette. Features of aortic transection on CXR include:

(a) Widened (>8 cm) superior mediastinum
(b) Superior thoracic cage fractures, including the 1st to 3rd ribs, sternum and scapula
(c) Obliteration of the aortic knob
(d) Left pleural effusion, hemothorax or apical pleural cap
(e) Deviation of the esophagus (nasogastric tube) and trachea (endotracheal tube) to the right
(f) Displacement of the left hilum downward
(g) Widening of the paratracheal and paraspinal stripe

Computed Tomography (CT) Angiography

It is used for definitive diagnosis of aortic transection and can also demonstrate associated orthopedic and thoracic injuries sustained during the trauma. Typical features of aortic transection on CT scan include:

(a) Disruption of the aortic lumen
(b) Extravasation of radioopaque contrast
(c) Periaortic hematoma

Patients with traumatic aortic rupture are managed according to the key principles of Advanced Trauma Life Support (ATLS), including airway, breathing and circulation. In some patients, it may be necessary to first treat "more" life-threatening injuries, such as pulmonary or cerebral trauma, before managing the aortic transection. If this is necessary, strict blood pressure control (maintaining systolic arterial pressure <110 mmHg) is required to reduce the risk of aortic rupture.

Traditionally, aortic transection is treated surgically by resecting the disrupted aorta and implanting an interposition graft through a left thoracotomy. This can either be performed using a "clamp and sew" technique or with the aid of a Gott shunt, left heart bypass or complete cardiopulmonary bypass. More recently, fluoroscopically guided endovascular stent grafting of the thoracic aorta is being increasingly used for the acute and delayed treatment of aortic transection. If the landing zone for the stent graft requires occlusion of the left subclavian artery, concomitant left common carotid-subclavian artery bypass may be required.

Discussion

Aortic transection is a life-threatening cardiothoracic surgical emergency. Although many patients do not present with any clinical features of aortic injury, it should be suspected in all patients with a history of deceleration injury during a road traffic accident and in all those with superior thoracic cage fractures. Contrast-enhanced spiral CT of the thorax is the investigation of choice for these patients to demonstrate the nature of the aortic trauma and any concomitant injuries.

Surgery or endovascular stent grafting should be performed immediately, unless other life-threatening injuries demand more urgent treatment. In patients with polytrauma, the use of endovascular stenting or surgery using low-dose systemic heparin is beneficial. Paraplegia and renal ischemia are the most serious complications of aortic transection and subsequent intervention.

Key Points

1. Aortic transection occurs following severe deceleration injury, usually associated with a road traffic accident.
2. Patients who reach hospital alive with aortic transection usually only have intimal and medial disruption. The adventitial layer, along with the surrounding mediastinal tissues, provides aortic luminal continuity.
3. Computed tomography angiography provides diagnostic imaging to delineate the nature of the aortic disruption and other associated injuries.
4. Treatment of other life-threatening injuries (such as pulmonary or cerebral trauma) may be required before definitive surgery or endovascular stenting of the aortic transection. In these patients, strict blood pressure control is required.
5. Immediate surgery or endovascular stenting is otherwise required for definitive treatment.

Chapter 9
Plastic Surgery Emergencies

Samer Saour and Pari-Naz Mohanna

Introduction

Plastic surgery embodies the importance of a scientific specialty requiring an artistic nature to result in excellent cosmetic and functional outcome for patients. As such, the importance of early diagnosis, with expeditious referral and treatment to centers of excellence is mandatory. Plastic surgical emergencies can be managed in general hospitals, but the level of expertise is not as great as that in centers of excellence, and hence urgent plastic surgical opinion should always be sought in such clinical cases.

Junior doctors will very rarely manage these emergencies themselves, however they should be acutely aware of initial steps in management, pending review by senior doctors. Conditions such as necrotizing fasciitis and compartment syndrome may be seen in all hospital wards. Urgent recognition, followed by emergency treatment and referral are essential for optimal outcome. Specific to plastic surgery, knowledge of the management of amputated parts, as well as

S. Saour, MB, BCh, BAO, MRCS, M.Sc. (✉)
P.-N. Mohanna, M.B.B.S., B.Sc., M.D., FRCS (plast)
Department of Plastic and Reconstructive Surgery,
Guy's and St. Thomas's NHS Foundation Trust, London, UK
e-mail: ssaour@hotmail.com

I. Shergill et al. (eds.), *Surgical Emergencies in Clinical Practice*, 161
DOI 10.1007/978-1-4471-2876-2_9,
© Springer-Verlag London 2013

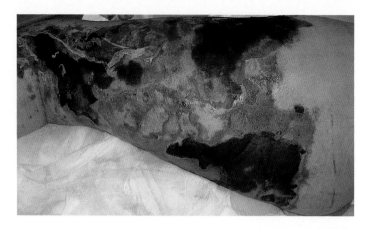

FIGURE 9.1 Necrotizing Fasciitis of the anterior and lateral abdominal wall extending to the chest and axilla. There is extensive erythema and fixed staining with areas of full thickness necrosis (black eschar)

their storage in the correct manner is mandatory, for satisfactory cosmetic and functional outcome. The final decision for surgery should be made by a senior doctor, ideally a Plastic Surgery Consultant.

Clinical Case Scenario 1: Necrotizing Fasciitis

Case Presentation

A 65 year old diabetic man was admitted with fever, chills and worsening cellulitis of his abdominal wall, 10 days following a punch biopsy of a lesion. The cellulitis had rapidly spread from the site of the biopsy to involve the anterior and lateral abdominal walls, spreading to the chest and axilla within 14 h (Fig. 9.1).

Key Features of History and Examination

Necrotizing Fasciitis (NF) is a clinical diagnosis and a life threatening condition.

History

NF tends to begin with constitutional symptoms of fever and chills. After 2–3 days, erythema is noted, and supralesional vesiculation or bullae formation ensues. Serosanguineous fluid may drain from the affected area. Necrotizing fasciitis may develop after skin biopsy; at needle puncture sites in those using illicit drugs; and after episodes of frostbite, chronic venous leg ulcers, open bone fractures, insect bites, surgical wounds, and skin abscesses. However, in many cases, no association with such factors can be made. NF may also occur in the setting of diabetes mellitus, surgery, trauma, or infectious processes.

Examination

Findings in NF may include all or some of the following clinical signs. A rapidly advancing erythema with painless ulcers appearing as the infection spreads along the fascial planes. A black necrotic eschar may be evident at the borders of the affected areas. Metastatic cutaneous plaques may occur. Septicemia is typical and leads to severe systemic toxicity and rapid death unless appropriately treated. In individuals with diabetes, crepitus is often evident, as are nonclostridial anaerobic infections. Purpura with or without bullae formation, occasionally with a lack of cutaneous erythema and heat, may be found, which does not preclude the diagnosis of NF.

Although the following features can occur with cellulitis, they are suggestive of NF:

- Rapid progression
- Poor therapeutic response
- Blistering necrosis
- Cyanosis
- Extreme local tenderness
- High temperature
- Tachycardia
- Hypotension
- Altered level of consciousness

Principles of Acute Management

Laboratory Studies

Laboratory tests, along with appropriate imaging studies, may facilitate the diagnosis of necrotizing fasciitis. Although the laboratory parameters may vary in a given clinical setting, the following may be associated with necrotizing fasciitis:

- WBC > 14,000/μL.
- Blood urea >15 mg/mL.
- Serum sodium <135 mmol/L.

Imaging Studies

Standard radiographs are of little value unless free air is depicted, as with gas-forming infections. MRI or CT scan delineation of the extent of NF may be useful in directing rapid surgical debridement

Other Tests

Excisional deep skin biopsy may be helpful in diagnosing and identifying the causative organisms. Cultures of the affected tissue obtained at initial debridement may be helpful. Gram staining of the exudate may provide a clue as to whether a type I or type II infection is present; the type influences the antibiotic therapy

Medical Therapy

This is a life threatening condition with a very high mortality rate. Management should occur within a multidisciplinary team setting. Ideally, the patient should be managed in an intensive care unit where hemodynamic parameters can be closely monitored. They will require;

1. Aggressive fluid resuscitation to offset acute renal failure and shock
2. Broad spectrum antibiotics are started, usually Clindamycin and Imipenem. This should be discussed with a microbiologist and may need to be changed when the gram stain/cultures have been reported
3. ITU supportive therapy with ventilation, inotropes and dialysis is also needed

Surgical Care

Once the diagnosis of NF is made, immediate surgical debridement is necessary. Surgical debridement and evaluations should be repeated almost on a daily basis until further tissue necrosis stops and the growth of fresh viable tissue is observed. If a limb or organ is involved, amputation may be necessary because of irreversible necrosis and gangrene or because of overwhelming toxicity.

These resultant wounds are best managed using a negative pressure dressing and once the tissue necrosis has stopped and the wounds are granulating they can be covered with a split skin graft.

Discussion

NF is a life threatening infection involving the superficial fascia and subcutaneous tissue. There are two types;

Type 1 involves mixed anaerobes and is usually seen in the vulnerable – young, old, immunosuppressed. It is usually an opportunistic infection

Type 2 involves Group A β-hemolytic *Streptococcus* (perfringens) infection which is the most common and usually affects previously fit individuals

Mortality rate is up to 50% with an often delayed presentation. There is no accepted classification system for necrotizing soft tissue infections. It is usually described on the basis of the tissue planes affected, the extent of invasion, anatomical site and causative pathogens. Deep soft tissue infections are classified either as necrotizing fasciitis or necrotizing myositis.

Key Learning Points

1. NF is a life threatening condition with a mortality rate of 50% often with a delayed presentation.
2. Early review by an experienced Doctor is essential.
3. Patients should be managed within a multidisciplinary team.
4. The mainstream of treatment involves ITU support, IV antibiotics and aggressive early surgical debridement of the affected area.
5. Surgical debridement must be repeated on a daily basis until the NF is under control.

Clinical Case Scenario 2: Pyogenic Flexor Tenosynovitis

Case Presentation

A 23 year old right hand dominant carpenter presented to the emergency department with a swollen and painful right index finger following a laceration with a Stanley knife 7 days earlier. He presented with a painful, swollen and stiff finger (Fig. 9.2) which had been gradually worsening.

Key Features of History and Examination

History

Patients with Pyogenic Flexor Tenosynovitis (PFT) can present at any time following a penetrating injury. They often complain of pain, swelling, redness and stiffness in the affected finger as well as accompanying fever.

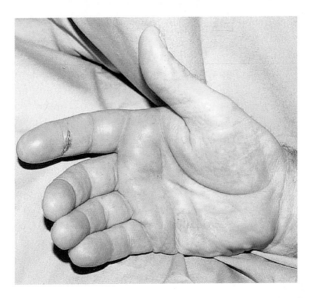

FIGURE 9.2 Pyogenic Flexor Tenosynovitis of the right index finger showing a laceration over the middle phalanx, fusiform swelling and erythema

Examination

Physical examination reveals Kanaval signs of flexor tendon sheath infection, which are (1) finger held in slight flexion, (2) fusiform swelling, (3) tenderness along the flexor tendon sheath, and (4) pain with passive extension of the digit. However, Kanaval signs may be absent in some patients, such as those who have recently had antibiotics administered, early presentations and immunocompromised patients.

The differential diagnosis of flexor tenosynovitis includes the following:

Inflammatory (nonsuppurative) flexor tenosynovitis
Herpetic whitlow
Pyarthrosis
Gout
Dactylitis
Phalanx fracture
Arthritis

Principles of Acute Management

If PFT is suspected, it is important to keep the patient nil by mouth and urgently refer them to a Plastic Surgery Unit. The indication for surgical drainage includes history and physical examination consistent with acute or chronic flexor tenosynovitis. In certain circumstances when acute flexor tenosynovitis presents within the first 24 h of onset, medical management may initially be trialed. Prompt improvement of symptoms and physical findings must follow within the ensuing 12 h; otherwise, surgical intervention is necessary.

Laboratory Studies

1. If infection is suggested, culture of the suppurative synovial fluid is mandatory prior to commencing definitive antimicrobial treatment

   These cultures should include aerobic, anaerobic, fungal and acid-fast bacilli
2. Full Blood Count

   WBC count may be elevated in the presence of proximal infection or systemic involvement. WBC count is not elevated in nonsuppurative conditions

   WBC count is often not elevated in immunocompromised patients.
3. Erythrocyte sedimentation rate (ESR)

   Although nonspecific, the ESR is typically elevated in acute or chronic infections and may serve as a marker to follow resolution of an infection

   ESR may be elevated in cases of inflammatory FT as well
4. Rheumatoid Factor is useful if rheumatoid arthritis is a consideration

Imaging Studies

Obtain standard anteroposterior and lateral radiographs to rule out bony involvement or retained foreign body.

Medical Treatment

If a patient presents very early medical treatment may initially be used. This includes;

1. Broad spectrum intravenous antibiotics
2. Elevation
3. Physiotherapy – once PFT is under control

Surgical Treatment

Indications;

1. No response to medical treatment within 12–24 h
2. Late presentation
3. Immunocompromised or diabetic patients

Surgical Procedure

Closed tendon sheath irrigation is carried out. A proximal incision is made over the A1 pulley. In the digit, either a standard Brunner incision or a midaxial incision may be utilized. The distal incision is made over the region of the A5 pulley. An appropriate size feeding tube is inserted into the tendon sheath through the proximal incision. The sheath is copiously irrigated with a minimum of 500 mL of normal saline. The wounds are left open, a splint is applied and the hand is elevated, and empiric antibiotic coverage is started while awaiting culture results.

After 24–48 h the wounds are inspected. For persisting infection, repeat operative debridement may be required. Otherwise: the wounds should be left open to heal by secondary intention and physiotherapy should be commenced. The switch from IV to oral antibiotics should be based not only on the culture results but also on the clinical examination and patient's progress.

Discussion

PFT results from an infectious agent multiplying in the closed space of the flexor tendon sheath and culture-rich synovial fluid medium. Natural immune response mechanisms cause swelling and migration of inflammatory cells and mediators. The septic process and inflammatory reaction within the tendon sheath quickly interfere with the gliding mechanism, leading to adhesions and scarring. This can ultimately result in tendon necrosis, disruption of the tendon sheath, and digital contracture.

The most common organisms responsible for disease include *Staphylococcus aureus* and *β-hemolytic Streptococcus*. If the initial injury was caused by an animal bite *Pasteurella multocida* should be suspected and if a human bite *Eikenella corrodens* or *Anaerobes*.

Key Learning Points

1. Clinical examination is the hallmark of diagnosis.
2. Kanaval signs of flexor tendon sheath infection are (1) finger held in slight flexion, (2) fusiform swelling, (3) tenderness along the flexor tendon sheath, and (4) pain with passive extension of the digit.
3. Kanavel's four cardinal signs may not all be present during the early stages of the disease, in the immunocompromised and in diabetics.
4. With early presentation medical management may be trialed however. prompt improvement of symptoms and physical findings must follow within the ensuing 12 h, otherwise, surgical intervention is necessary.
5. Surgical washout is the mainstay of treatment

Clinical Case Scenario 3: Digit Amputation

Case Presentation

A 40 year old right hand dominant factory worker presented to the emergency department following an accident with an industrial press. He suffered total amputation of his dominant index finger at the level of the proximal interphalangeal joint. The accident occurred at 9 a.m. and the patient and amputated part arrived by ambulance to the emergency department at 10 a.m.

Key Features of History and Examination

History

An adequate history is essential and should include the age of the patient, hand dominance, occupation, hobbies, the mechanism, time, and place of injury, condition of the injured part, general condition of the patient and smoking history.

1. The mechanism of amputation is important with sharp injuries having a much better chance of successful replantation than those caused by blunt crushing forces. The six mechanisms of amputation injury are;

    Sharp cut, as from a knife or meat slicer
    Dull cut, as from a saw or dull edge (e.g., fan blade)
    Cut with a narrow segment of crush injury, as from a punch press
    Cut and avulsion, as from a machine that causes partial amputation and subsequent reflexive withdrawal of the hand that completes the amputation
    Avulsion, as from a finger or a hand caught in an anchor rope or horse reins
    Crush avulsion, as from a machine (e.g., rollers) that crushes the limb then pulls the digits off

2. The time elapsed since injury and the method by which the amputated part has been stored are crucial. If the warm ischemia time is greater than 6 h for an amputation proximal to the carpus or 12 h for the digits, replantation is not usually recommended. In addition, if the cold ischemia time is greater than 12 h for a proximal amputation, replantation is not generally performed.

3. Ask about any old injuries to the affected hand.

4. Ask about the patient's pre-morbid condition. Negative prognostic factors include old age, peripheral vascular

disease, congestive heart failure, and diabetes mellitus with complications. In the surgeon's judgment, these factors may make replantation inadvisable.

5. Assess the patient's psychiatric history. If the amputation was self-inflicted, a psychiatric evaluation is recommended and replantation may not be advisable.

Examination

Perform a detailed examination of the hand and the amputated part to assess;

1. Location and level of amputation
2. Whether the injury is at a single or multiple levels
3. Whether single or multiple digits are amputated
4. Condition of the amputated part, including signs of avulsion or crush
5. Degree of tissue loss (skin, vessel, bone, nerve, tendon)
6. Amount of contamination
7. Thorough neurovascular examination of the extremity

Principles of Acute Management

The patient should be managed in accordance with the Advance Trauma Life Support (ATLS) protocol. Major life threatening injuries take precedence over replantation of an amputated digit. Once the patient is stable they should be transferred to a Plastic Surgery Unit.

Laboratory Studies

1. Hemoglobin and hematocrit
2. Type and cross-match 2–4 units of packed red blood cells if the patient's history suggests significant blood loss

Imaging Studies

Obtain posteroanterior, lateral, and oblique radiographs of the amputated part and stump.

Carefully assess for radiopaque foreign bodies

Comminution of the fracture implies a crush injury mechanism and is associated with soft-tissue trauma

If the joint is destroyed at the level of amputation, arthrodesis may be indicated resulting in a loss of joint function

If a crush injury is severe, a mosaic of fragments may preclude attempts at replantation

Other investigations are indicated by the patients age and associated medical history

Emergency Department Care

1. Control bleeding by applying direct pressure and elevating the limb
2. Ensure that the patient is covered for tetanus
3. Start prophylactic antibiotics. Common pathogens are *Staphylococcus aureus* and group A streptococci
4. Administer analgesia
5. Transfer patient and amputated part to a Plastic Surgery Unit

Correct Storage of the Amputated Part

The amputated part should be wrapped in moist (saline) gauze and placed in a sealed plastic bag. The sealed bag is placed in a container containing an ice-saline bath to maintain a temperature of 4°C (cold ischemia). The amputated part should never be placed directly onto the ice or into a hyper or hypotonic solution.

One hour of warm ischemia is equivalent to approximately 6 h of cold ischemia. Hence, cooling can markedly prolong the window of opportunity for replantation.

Replantation

This can be performed under a regional block or a general anesthetic. Two teams are required one preparing the amputated stump under tourniquet and magnification and the other the amputated part. The surgical sequence is as follows;

1. Debridement of the stump and the amputated part
2. Identification and tagging of arteries, veins, nerves and tendons
3. Bony stabilization
4. Extensor tendon repair
5. Flexor tendon repair
6. Arterial anastomosis
7. Venous anastomosis
8. Nerve repair
9. Skin closure; direct, flap or graft.

Post Operative Care

1. Splinting to immobilize and protect the replanted part
2. Frequent and careful monitoring of the vascular status of the replanted part; examining for color, turgor, temperature and capillary refill.
3. Keep patient warm and well hydrated
4. Administer adequate analgesia

General Discussion

Replantation is the reattachment of a part that has been completely amputated with no connection existing between the severed part and the patient. Revascularization is the repair of a part that has been incompletely amputated, with some of the soft tissues (e.g., skin, nerves, or tendons) remaining intact.

Bone, tendon, and skin can tolerate approximately 8–12 h of warm ischemia and as long as 24 h of cold ischemia. However, muscle necrosis after 6 h of warm ischemia or 12 h of cold ischemia. In general, amputated digits may tolerate 12 h of warm ischemia and 24 h of cold ischemia. Other major amputations tolerate 6 h of warm ischemia and 12 h of cold ischemia because of their larger muscle content. Excessive ischemia time reduces muscle function and can result in myoglobinuria on reperfusion,

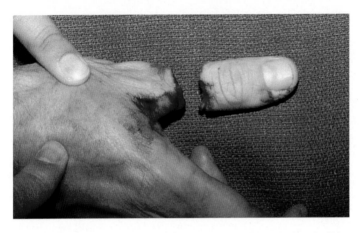

FIGURE 9.3 Sharp amputation of the right thumb at the level of the proximal phalanx

placing renal function at risk. More proximal amputations involving more muscle must therefore be treated quickly.

Patient selection for replantation is very important. Below are the indications and contraindication to replantation, which should be used as a guide. Even with these guides the decision to replant can be very difficult and must be made by a Senior Plastic Surgeon, ideally a Consultant.

Indications

Individual digit distal to the flexor digitorum superficialis tendon
Thumb (Fig. 9.3) and multiple digits
Amputation through the palm, wrist or forearm
Amputations in children

Contraindications

Severely crushed or mangled parts
Amputations at multiple levels

Amputations in patients with other major trauma or severe medical diseases

Amputations with prolonged warm ischemia

Five Key Learning Points

1. Manage patient according to the ATLS principles.
2. Ascertain timing and mechanism of injury.
3. The amputated part must be stored in the correct way and never directly on ice.
4. Promptly transfer the patient and the amputated part to a Plastic Surgery Unit.
5. The decision to perform a replantation should be made by a senior doctor ideally a Consultant Plastic Surgeon.

Clinical Case Scenario 4: Upper Limb Compartment Syndrome

Case Presentation

A 35 year old right handed mechanic presented to the emergency department following an engine falling onto his forearm. One hour after the accident he noticed started complaining of worsening pain and tightness in his forearm to the point where the pain was unbearable. He also noted numbness affecting the index and middle finger.

Key Features of History and Examination

Compartment syndrome (CS) is a clinical diagnosis.

History

Ascertain the patients hand dominance, occupation and hobbies. The onset of pain may have been preceded by trauma. High level of suspicion should be maintained in patients who suffer

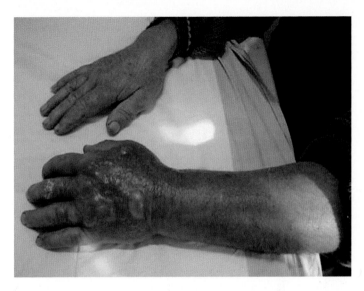

FIGURE 9.4 Compartment Syndrome of the left forearm and hand showing significant swelling and blisters

long bone fractures, high velocity injuries, high energy trauma or penetrating injuries. The pain is persistent, progressive, unrelieved by immobilization and out of proportion to the original injury. The patient may also describe a tense feeling in the extremity as well as diminished sensation and weakness.

Examination

The physical examination must be repeated to determine if signs have progressed. Comparison of the affected limb to the unaffected limb is useful (Fig. 9.4). There may be evidence of trauma. The pain is deep and is worsened by passive stretching of the muscles within the affected compartment. There may be diminished 2-point discrimination and vibration sense. The most important diagnostic physical finding is a firm, wooden feeling on deep palpation. Bullae may also be seen; however, so-called fracture blisters are common in the absence of CS. Late findings include pallor and loss of pulses. More importantly the presence of a pulse does not exclude the possibility of a CS. If muscle weakness is found the CS is very advanced.

Principles of Acute Management

The patient should be managed in accordance with the Advance Trauma Life Support (ATLS) protocol. If CS is suspected urgent referral to a Plastic Surgery Unit is essential.

Laboratory Studies

1. CK (creatine kinase) is used to determine the degree of muscle necrosis

   Serial CK measurements may show rising levels indicative of a developing CS

   High CK levels should alert the physician to possible rhabdomyolysis

2. Urea, creatinine and electrolytes are used to assess kidney function in cases of rhabdomyolysis
3. Complete blood cell count and coagulation studies
4. Urine analysis is used to determine myoglobin and CK levels

Imaging Studies

Imaging studies are usually not helpful in making the diagnosis of CS. However such studies are used in part to eliminate disorders in the differential diagnosis.

Diagnostic Procedures

Compartment pressures can be measured to support the diagnosis, but the diagnosis is essentially based on clinical findings. Compartment pressure of greater than 30 mmHg requires intervention.

Medical Therapy

1. Place the affected limb or limbs at the level of the heart. Elevation is contraindicated because it decreases arterial flow and narrows the arterial-venous pressure gradient.
2. Keep the patient well hydrated maintaining a urine output >1–2 mL/kg/h

Surgical Therapy

The treatment of choice for CS is early decompression with the goal of salvaging a functional extremity.

Decompression fasciotomy of the forearm is performed through a volar and dorsal approach. In the forearm, the volar, dorsal, and mobile wad compartments are interconnected. Therefore superficial fasciotomy is usually adequate to decompress the entire forearm. Forearm fasciotomy requires decompression from the wrist to mid arm using a curvilinear incision. This incision can be extended into the palm to release the carpal tunnel. Decompression of the hand is done through two dorsal incisions, one between the 1st and 2nd metacarpal bones and the second between the 4th and 5th metacarpals. Further incisions over the thenar and hypothenar muscles are also carried out.

Post Operative Care

Elevate the affected extremity for 24–48 h. If necrotic muscle develops this needs to be excised. Delayed primary closure of the skin can usually be accomplished at 5 days. If this is not possible a split skin graft should be applied.

General Discussion

CS occurs when the tissue pressure within a closed muscle compartment exceeds the perfusion pressure and results in muscle and nerve ischemia. The cycle of events leading to acute CS begins when the tissue pressure exceeds the venous pressure and impairs blood outflow. Lack of oxygenated blood and lack of waste product removal result in pain and decreased peripheral sensation secondary to nerve irritation. Late manifestations of CS include the absence of a distal pulse, hypoesthesia, and extremity paresis because the cycle of elevating tissue pressure eventually compromises arterial blood flow. If left untreated, the muscles and nerves within the compartment undergo necrosis, and a limb contracture, called a Volkmann contracture.

Five Key Learning Points

1. Compartment Syndrome is a clinical diagnosis
2. Compartment Syndrome should be suspected whenever significant pain occurs in an extremity after injury, especially if it is tense
3. Pain during passive stretching is one of the earliest clinical signs of Compartment Syndrome. Other symptoms include paraesthesia (sensory nerves affected first), paralysis, weakness and a tense limb. Pulselessness is a late sign and would indicate advanced Compartment Syndrome
4. Urgent referral to a Plastic Surgery Unit is essential
5. Urgent surgical decompression is a limb saving procedure

Clinical Case Scenario 5: Extravasation Injury

Case Presentation

A 35 year old woman with breast cancer was receiving a chemotherapeutic agent through a peripheral line. After half an hour she began to experience pain and swelling in the dorsum of her right hand. She alerted the nursing staff who immediately stopped the infusion.

Key Features of History and Examination

History

Pain at the intravenous site may be modest or severe, usually burning or stinging

Assess the extent of the extravasation;

- Site of the extravasation
- Type of agent used
- Concentration of the agent
- Dose of the agent
- Was there a delay in recognition and initiation of treatment
- Type of treatment initiated

Examination

There may be erythema, swelling, tenderness, and lack of blood return from the cannula

Local blistering is indicative of at least a partial-thickness skin injury. There may also be mottling and darkening of the skin and firm induration

When the full thickness of the skin is damaged, the surface may appear very white and cold with no capillary return and later may develop a dry, black eschar (Fig. 9.5)

Ulceration is not usually evident until 1 or 2 weeks after the injury when the eschar sloughs to reveal the underlying ulcer (Fig. 9.6)

Principles of Acute Management

On suspecting extravasation stop the injection/infusion immediately

Aspirate any residual drug and blood through the cannula to remove as much of the drug from the site as possible and minimize tissue damage

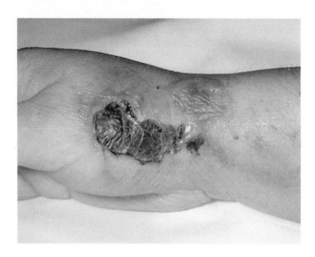

FIGURE 9.5 Extravasation injury of the right anatomical snuff box, showing erythema, blistering and black eschar formation

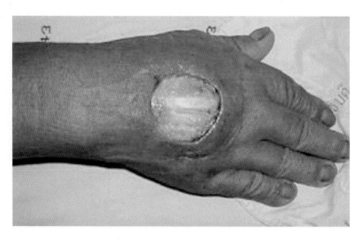

FIGURE 9.6 Ulceration of the dorsum of the right hand following extravasation injury. The extensor tendons are exposed

Remove the cannula and mark round the extravasated area with a marker pen to provide a baseline for monitoring the extent of the extravasation

The decision to washout the area depends on the agent and its toxicity. Toxic agents include chemotherapeutic drugs, noradrenaline, dopamine, phenytoin, albumin and solutions that contain hypertonic dextrose. If any of these agents have been used or if there are any skin changes, the area should be washed out

This can be done under local anesthetic using the Gault protocol. Hyaluronidase is injected into the area of extravasation. Four small stab incisions are made around the zone of extravasation injury and a thorough flush out of the extravasation space with Normal Saline is carried out thought a blunt ended cannula.

The area is then dressed and elevated to help reduce the swelling. The area is reviewed on a daily until it has healed.

General Discussion

Extravasation occurs when there is non-intentional leakage of infused fluid into the surrounding tissue, which subsequently leads to tissue damage and skin necrosis.

The key is Prevention. Various *strategies* have been introduced to try and reduce the risk of extravasation injury in preterm neonates:

Siting of central lines for the administration of total parenteral nutrition and infusions which contain glucose in concentrations greater than 10%

Hourly recording of observations at the cannulation site for signs of edema, firmness or discoloration

Securing the cannulae with a transparent dressing to allow unobstructed visibility at the insertion site

The use of pressure sensitive infusion pumps

Five Key Learning Points

1. Early recognition is important
2. Stop the infusion straight away and aspirate as much fluid as possible through the intravenous cannula before taking it out
3. Seek senior help, and/or refer to a Plastic Surgeon
4. If a toxic agent has been used or if there are any skin changes, the area should be washed out urgently with Normal saline
5. Daily reviews are then needed to observe for any complications

Further Reading

Simonart T, Simonart JM, Derdelinckx I, et al. Value of standard laboratory tests for the early recognition of group A beta-hemolytic streptococcal necrotizing fasciitis. Clin Infect Dis. 2001;32(1):E9–12.

Kanavel A. Infections of the hand. 4th ed. Philadelphia: Lea & Febiger; 1921.

Neviaser R. Closed tendon sheath irrigation for pyogenic flexor tenosynovitis. J Hand Surg [Am]. 1978;3:462–6.

Komatsu S, Tamai S. Successful replantation of a completely cut-off thumb: case report. Plast Reconstr Surg. 1968;42:374–7.

Malt RA, McKhann C. Replantation of severed arms. JAMA. 1964;189:716.

von Volkmann R. Veilletzungen und Krankenheiten der Berwegungsorgane. In: von Pithe F, Billroth T, editors. Handbuch der Allgemeinen und Speziellen Chirurgs. Zweiter Band, Zweiter Abteilung, Abschmitt V, Ersted haft. Stuttgart: Verlag von Ferdinand Enke; 1882. p. 234–920.

Gault DT. Extravasation injuries. Br J Plast Surg. 1993;46(2): 91–6.

Chapter 10
Neurosurgery Emergencies

Alan W. Hewitt and David Choi

Introduction

There are very few dedicated neurosurgical departments in the country, and as such, referrals from a wide geographical area are common. Initial management, therefore, of such emergencies is often done in general hospitals, often under the care of general surgical or trauma and orthopedic specialties, which may not have any specialist knowledge of neurosurgical conditions. These facts may result in sub-optimum care for patients who are at risk of life-threatening conditions.

Importantly, it should be remembered that the skull is essentially a closed space, and, as such, there is no room for expansion in this space. Those patients who initially appear to have a simple head injury may have a sudden change in clinical

A.W. Hewitt, M.A., FRCS (SN)(✉)
Department of Spine Surgery, James Cook University Hospital,
Middlesbrough, Teeside, UK
e-mail: alanwhewitt@doctors.org.uk

D. Choi, M.A., MBChB, FRCS, Ph.D.
Department of Neurosurgery, Institute of Neurology and Neurosurgery,
University College London, London, UK

Department of Neurosurgery, The National Hospital for Neurology
and Neurosurgery, London, UK

I. Shergill et al. (eds.), *Surgical Emergencies in Clinical Practice*, 185
DOI 10.1007/978-1-4471-2876-2_10,
© Springer-Verlag London 2013

condition, especially if underlying brain conditions are not recognized or inappropriately treated.

This chapter outlines the main neurosurgical emergencies which junior trainees should be fully aware of how to diagnose, initially manage, and then appropriately transfer to regional neurosurgical center for optimal patient outcome. The mere fact that the brain and spinal cord are made of cells which are generally unable to regenerate, should they become irreversibly injured, should highlight the trainee to the importance of early diagnosis and early treatment, with expeditious and appropriate transfer to specialist neurosurgical center.

Clinical Case Scenario 1: Diffuse Brain Injury

Case Presentation

A 26-year-old man is riding his motorcycle on a main road when he skids, colliding with a tree. On arrival, the ambulance crew finds he has a diminished conscious level with signs of head injury. Oxygen and cervical spine immobilization are administered, and he is transferred to the nearby accident and emergency department (A&E) with en route call to alert the trauma team. On arrival in A&E, the trauma team performs ATLS assessment and resuscitation. There is no evidence of noisy breathing or shock but his conscious level is such that his best responses are flexion (decorticate) to painful stimulus, utters incomprehensible sounds, with no eye opening. Pupils are equal and reactive with symmetrical limb responses. He is intubated immediately by the anesthetist and ventilated with oxygen, and a primary survey is completed including chest and pelvic X-ray. CT of the brain and cervical spine is obtained without delay (Fig. 10.1) and the leader of the trauma team contacts the regional neurosurgical on call registrar by telephone. The images show no focal hematoma, and the diagnosis is severe diffuse brain injury. No emergency surgery is required and transfer is arranged to the neurosurgical ITU.

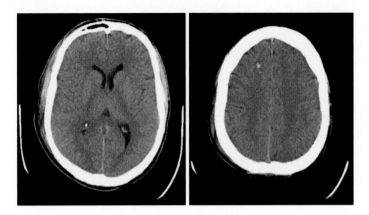

FIGURE 10.1 Diffuse brain injury Axial CT. Note that even in this severe brain injury, the image on the *left* is not significantly abnormal. The higher slice shows small petechial hemorrhages in the right frontal lobe which are commonly seen in this type of injury

Key Features of History and Examination

Initial assessment uses the ATLS approach common to all trauma patients. Certain points are particularly important in brain injury.

- Mechanism – brain injury causes approximately a quarter of all trauma deaths in Britain, and around half are caused by road accidents. The energy level involved informs as to the likely severity and type of brain injury. A high-energy mechanism is likely to result in more severe primary brain injury, that is, when the brain is injured severely at the moment of impact.
- Immediate priority is recognition of the unsafe or occluded airway, recognition of hypoventilation or shock, and associated injuries threatening breathing or circulation as these are potentially treatable factors which will cause exacerbation of the injury, that is, secondary brain injury.
- It is essential to accurately assess and record conscious level, using the Glasgow Coma Scale (GCS – see Table 10.1), and any asymmetry of limb responses and papillary responses as

TABLE 10.1 Glasgow Coma Scale (GCS)

Assessment area	Score
Best motor response (*M*)	
Obeys commands	6
Localizes pain	5
Normal flexion (withdrawal)	4
Abnormal flexion (decorticate)	3
Extension (decerebrate)	2
None (flaccid)	1
Verbal response (*V*)	
Orientated	5
Confused conversation	4
Inappropriate single words	3
Incomprehensible sounds	2
None	1
Eye opening (*E*)	
Spontaneous	4
To speech	3
To pain	2
None	1

GCS score $= (E + M + V)$; best possible score $= 15$; worst possible score $= 3$

part of the initial assessment and prior to intubation. The conscious level is the most important indicator of the severity of brain injury. Pupillary dilatation may indicate brain herniation with compression of the oculomotor nerve which may occur in severe injuries. A unilateral dilated pupil is a reliable indicator of which side of the brain is affected when it is caused by a focal lesion such as a hematoma.

- Each assessment area of the GCS must be recorded individually – motor response, verbal response, and eye opening – rather than the total score. The motor response is the most important guide to the severity of brain injury in most cases, and this essential information must not be embedded within a total score.

- History of conscious level on the scene and subsequent deterioration or improvement will indicate information as to the severity and type of injury. A lucid interval is indicative of a less severe primary brain injury which, if followed by deterioration, may become a severe secondary brain injury.
- Assessment of the safety of the airway includes the conscious level. An adequate sensorium is required to protect the airway; therefore, an apparently clear airway is not safe if the conscious level is severely reduced and intubation is necessary.

Principles of Acute Management

Brain injury may be classified as primary – that which occurs at the moment of impact – and secondary – that which complicates the initial injury. The main principle of immediate management is to minimize the secondary brain injury. Primary brain injury may be prevented or minimized, for example, by road safety initiatives or vehicle design, but is not treatable.

- Good ATLS management is key, as hypoventilation, obstructed breathing, and shock contributes rapidly to secondary brain injury, morbidity, and death.
- The conscious level and particularly motor response is the most important indicator of severity, and this may be classified as mild, moderate, or severe.
- Severe brain injury, when GCS is 8 or less, is associated with inadequate consciousness to protect the airway, so intubation is mandatory for all patients with potentially survivable injuries.
- Following initial resuscitation, CT of the head and C-spine should be performed without delay. This will indicate whether there is a focal injury, for example, acute subdural hematoma, extradural hematoma, or intracerebral hematoma (contusion), which might require surgical resection, or a diffuse injury as in this case.
- All patients with a significant brain injury should be discussed with the regional neurosurgery team.

Discussion

In the "golden hour" following trauma, it is coordination of good ATLS care which is key. This may be provided by paramedics, A&E staff, and dedicated trauma teams. Systems must be developed to allow the A, B, C, D, and E of trauma care to be delivered in a consistent and coordinated manner. In a modern hospital, this will involve an ATLS-trained team performing simultaneous assessment and management of each of these aspects of care, but if that is not possible, then they must be worked through in that order of priority.

Following resuscitation, CT will allow the neurosurgeon to identify those patients who require urgent surgery for traumatic lesions causing mass effect. Many patients who have severe diffuse brain injury with no specific surgical lesion will also require transfer to the neurosurgical ITU. This will allow invasive monitoring of intracranial pressure by a transducing probe which is placed in the parenchyma or ventricle of the brain, and protocol-guided, coordinated specialist ITU care which aims to minimize secondary brain injury. There is evidence that those patients with severe diffuse injuries who are managed in a dedicated neurosciences center have better eventual outcome than those managed in general ITU. It is as yet unknown which aspects of management produce this difference in outcome [1].

Key Points

1. Secondary brain injury is potentially treatable, and effective ATLS trauma care is the most important factor during the "golden hour."
2. The key aspects of emergency neurological assessment are the GCS with assessment of the pupils and asymmetry of limb responses. This indicates the severity of the injury and may indicate if there is a mass lesion in one side of the brain. It is essential to record the motor, verbal, and eye opening components of the GCS separately rather than just the total score.

3. When the GCS is 8 or less, immediate intubation is usually required.
4. CT of the brain and cervical spine should be obtained without delay which will allow the neurosurgeon to identify those patients requiring emergency surgery.
5. Severely brain-injured patients who do not require emergency surgery also often require transfer to the neurosurgical center for specialist care in ITU.

Clinical Case Scenario 2: Subarachnoid Hemorrhage

Case Presentation

A 55-year-old woman presents to accident and emergency department with a sudden onset of headache. It is the worst headache she has ever experienced and felt as though she had been struck on the back of the head. It occurred while she was in the classroom working as a school teacher. She reports no loss of consciousness but she vomited repeatedly. One hour later, the headache is continuing and she is very nauseated. She now complains of double vision and prefers dim light. Her past medical history includes hypertension and migraine, and she is an ex-smoker. On examination, she has photophobia and neck stiffness but is afebrile. The GCS is 14/15 (obeying commands, orientated, eye opening to speech). Examination of cranial nerves reveals that the right eye is not abducting fully and the diplopia occurs on looking to the right. CT of the brain confirms subarachnoid hemorrhage (Fig. 10.2).

Key Features of History and Examination

The symptom of sudden onset of headache always raises suspicion of subarachnoid hemorrhage.

• The headache typically occurs without warning but may occasionally be preceded by a headache of lesser severity

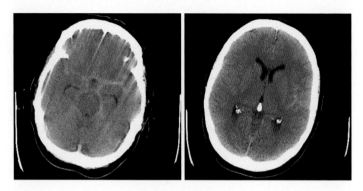

FIGURE 10.2 Subarachnoid hemorrhage non-contrast axial CT. The image on the *left* is at the level of the basal cisterns and clearly shows hyperdensity (blood) filling the basal cisterns, extending into the Sylvian fissures, and surrounding the brainstem. This image is clearly diagnostic of subarachnoid hemorrhage. The mild dilatation of the temporal horns of the ventricles in the left image is very common. The image on the *right* is a higher cut from the same study which demonstrates that there is not significant hydrocephalus or ventricular blood load

(sentinel headache). It may occur during coitus or wake the patient from sleep.

- Collapse is common and many patients (around one-third) may present in coma.
- Vomiting occurs in most cases but may be absent.
- Neck stiffness and photophobia usually occurs.
- It is uncommon in children but may occur at any age. There is a slight peak in late middle age with slight female preponderance.
- There is a strong association with polycystic kidney disease and Marfan's syndrome and a weak genetic factor in patients without any such syndrome. The great majority of cases are sporadic.
- For sporadic cases, smoking and hypertension are weakly associated risk factors but identifiable risk factors are often absent.

- A past history of migraine or other headache should never distract from the suspicion of subarachnoid hemorrhage.
- Neurological examination must establish the GCS, and each aspect – motor, verbal, and eye opening responses – must be recorded separately.
- Cranial nerve examination should include careful assessment of eye movements. Oculomotor nerve palsy may occur as a result of direct contact with an aneurysm arising close to that nerve (commonly posterior communicating artery aneurysm) or may occur as a result of brain herniation for those patients with impaired conscious level. Abducent nerve palsy may occur without any direct structural contact, as it is a long, delicate nerve which is susceptible to stretching. This may occur particularly when hydrocephalus develops.
- Examination of the limbs may reveal hemiparesis or monoparesis (weakness of a single limb).

Principles of Acute Management

It is essential to establish the diagnosis without delay and refer to neurosurgery. This enables treatment to prevent rebleeding as well as detection and treatment of complications, especially hydrocephalus and vasospasm with delayed ischemia.

- CT should be obtained promptly for all patients with clinical suspicion of subarachnoid hemorrhage. When obtained within 48 h of the hemorrhage, it has 95% sensitivity in confirming the diagnosis.
- When CT is negative, all patients require lumbar puncture (unless contraindicated) if there is clinical suspicion of subarachnoid hemorrhage.
- Lumbar puncture with analysis of CSF by spectrophotometry is the gold standard. Spectrophotometry for the presence of bilirubin is essential to differentiate between subarachnoid hemorrhage and blood from the trauma of the lumbar puncture. Bilirubin is formed in vivo in CSF by enzyme-dependent breakdown of blood in approximately

6 h, but is not formed following traumatic lumbar puncture. It should be confirmed with the lab that spectrophotometry can be performed before performing the lumbar puncture. Older methods of attempting to differentiate between subarachnoid hemorrhage and traumatic tap such as comparison of red cell counts in three CSF samples are unreliable and should not be used.

- Lumbar puncture should be performed between 12 h and 2 weeks of the onset of symptoms. When performed in this interval, the reported sensitivity is 100%. Many surgeons consider that delay of greater than 1 week could risk false negative error.
- History of headache of other cause, for example, migraine, must not distract from appropriate investigation if current symptoms raise suspicion of subarachnoid hemorrhage, nor should investigation results such as ECG changes which may occur in subarachnoid hemorrhage.
- If diagnosis is missed because lumbar puncture is not performed when it is required, a likely consequence is that the patient will suffer a further preventable hemorrhage in the subsequent 6 months with a high risk of mortality.
- Once diagnosed, all cases should be referred to neurosurgery by telephone without delay. The clinical details must be accurately explained. For patients in good grade (conscious and without disabling neurological deficit), usual management will include bed rest, oxygen, intravenous infusion with 3 l of 0.9% saline per day with potassium replacement, nimodipine 60 mg 4 hourly by mouth, laxatives, and analgesia with paracetamol and codeine. Those patients in poor grade require admission to critical care.
- Nimodipine is a calcium channel antagonist which has been shown to improve rates of vasospasm and delayed ischemia which may complicate subarachnoid hemorrhage.
- Daily U&E is necessary as hypokalemia and hyponatremia are very common in the metabolic aftermath of subarachnoid hemorrhage. Hypokalemia results from the profound stress response whereas sodium is usually lost as a result of cerebral salt wasting. Both are treated by intravenous

replacement with fluid; fluid restriction is generally contraindicated in subarachnoid hemorrhage.

- All patients in good grade will be transferred to the neurosurgical unit. Imaging (CT angiography) will be used to
  confirm that a cerebral aneurysm has caused the hemorrhage, and treatment (endovascular coiling or craniotomy
  and clipping) to occlude the aneurysm will be offered on the
  next available list with the aim of prevention of rebleeding.
- In the event of deterioration of conscious level, CT is
  obtained, and if hydrocephalus is present, this may be treated
  by surgical placement of an external ventricular drain.

Discussion

Spontaneous subarachnoid hemorrhage is due to ruptured
cerebral aneurysm in approximately 80% of cases. This may be
fatal in approximately one-third of cases. Those who survive
without treatment would face the likelihood of rebleeding with
a risk of approximately 50% in 6 months with high mortality
rates. Once diagnosed, however, the aneurysm can usually be
occluded without complication, and a majority of patients
admitted to the neurosurgical unit in good grade have a good
outcome. A potentially potent cause of avoidable adverse outcome is therefore missed diagnosis. The key to emergency management is early diagnosis and discussion with neurosurgery.
The diagnosis is often easy, but problems arise when CT is
negative and there are distracting factors in the presentation. It
is essential that lumbar puncture is performed with spectrophotometry analysis of the CSF in these cases. In case of any doubt,
neurosurgery should be consulted.

Key Points

1. The typical symptoms of subarachnoid hemorrhage are
   sudden severe headache with vomiting, neck stiffness, and
   photophobia, but remember that the key feature is the
   onset. Any sudden onset headache raises suspicion.

2. All patients with clinical suspicion of subarachnoid hemorrhage must have CT. If CT is negative, this should be followed by lumbar puncture at least 12 h and less than 1 week following the onset of symptoms. If there is delayed presentation, contraindication to lumbar puncture or any other concerned neurosurgery should be consulted.

3. Clinical findings of conscious level and focal neurological deficit allow the hemorrhage to be graded by the neurosurgeon, which will influence management, so this information must be accurately recorded and clearly communicated in the referral.

4. Management following diagnosis will be guided by neurosurgery and will consist of oxygen, intravenous saline, oral nimodipine, bed rest, analgesia and daily electrolyte testing, or admission to critical care if necessary.

5. Early transfer to the neurosurgical unit will usually be appropriate. Imaging for cerebral aneurysm will then be performed, and, if present, it will then be occluded by coiling or clipping to prevent rebleeding.

Clinical Case Scenario 3: Cauda Equina Syndrome

Case Presentation

A 32-year-old plumber has a chronic history of back pain. One week before admission, he develops sudden sharp back pain on moving which develops over hours into an agonizing electric pain which extends down his left leg and into the lateral part of his foot. He has suffered from sciatica in the past and self-medicates in the expectation of spontaneous improvement. The day before admission, the pain spreads to involve both buttocks but is no more severe. The morning of admission he notices that the pain is actually less severe, but he has numbness affecting his buttocks, anal region, and penis. In the afternoon, he becomes incontinent of urine and attends the accident and emergency department. On examination, he has

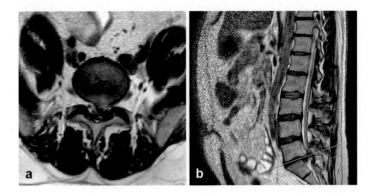

FIGURE 10.3 Sagittal and axial T2 MRI showing a large disc prolapse which is causing severe central and left-sided cauda equina compression

dribbling incontinence of urine. A urinary catheter is placed with 1,100 ml of urine filling the bag. He does not feel the catheter. Positive straight leg raise is present bilaterally, although his sciatica is now less severe than before. Sensation is markedly reduced to pinprick but present to fine touch on the lateral border of the left foot, the back of the left leg, the back of the right thigh, and both buttocks. Rectal examination reveals diminished sensation and reduced anal tone. Power is apparently intact in all muscle groups. Reflexes are absent at both ankles but normal at the knees. Plantar responses are downgoing. A clinical diagnosis of cauda equina syndrome is made and MRI of the lumbosacral spine is obtained urgently (Fig. 10.3).

Key Features of History and Examination

History and examination must establish the diagnosis, duration, and severity of the syndrome.

The cauda equina syndrome occurs when multiple nerve roots in the lumbar spine (the cauda equina) are simultaneously crushed by a central disc prolapse. The features of the cauda equina syndrome are those of loss of function of the affected roots. Therefore, the key to diagnosis of the syndrome

TABLE 10.2 Function of the nerve roots consisting the cauda equina

Root	L4	L5	S1	S2/3/4
Sensory loss	Knee, medial Lower leg	Dorsum of foot, big toe	Lateral foot	Back of leg, buttocks, perineum
Motor loss (Main)	Inversion of foot	Foot drop (often severe)	Plantar flexion and eversion of foot (may be mild)	Bladder, bowel, and sexual function
Reflex loss	Knee jerk	None	Ankle jerk	

is to have a working knowledge of the function of the nerve roots potentially involved and knowledge of how to recognize when these functions are lost.

A working knowledge of only a few roots is required (Table 10.2) because such disc prolapses do not tend to occur except at the lowest levels in the lumbar spine: L5/S1 and L4/5 levels. Disc prolapse causing cauda equina syndrome rarely occurs above L3/4 level.

- A complete cauda equina syndrome at L5/S1 level affects S1, S2, S3, and S4 roots bilaterally, that is, all roots below L5
- A complete cauda equina syndrome at L4/5 affects L5, S1, S2, S3, and S4 roots bilaterally, that is, all roots below L5
- Note that the prominent features are sensory symptoms with incontinence rather than motor deficits affecting the limbs. Severe cauda equina syndrome at L5/S1 often only causes a motor deficit of plantar flexion which may be mild, whereas at L4/5, there will also be footdrop which is usually more severe. Paraparesis is not a feature of cauda equina syndrome, although L4, L5 and S1 deficits can also cause weakness of hip extension and knee flexion.
- Where motor signs occur, they are lower motor neuron. Reflexes are absent at the ankles. Brisk reflexes are not a feature of cauda equina syndrome and imply that the pathology affects the thoracic or cervical spinal cord, brain, or both, and investigations should be planned accordingly.

- Typically, nerve roots affected by disc prolapse first produce pain in the dermatomal distribution, followed by paresthesia and finally numbness. This is understood as a progression from abnormal function to loss of function.
- The duration of symptoms must be noted as well as rate of any deterioration.
- Incontinence with impaired sensation is a cardinal feature. This is important because urinary retention is not uncommon during an attack of simple sciatica due to pain inhibition of bladder emptying rather than a deficit of the cauda equina. If there is numbness of buttocks or perineum, painless urinary retention, or inability to feel the catheter, occurring with or after sciatica, this is very suggestive of cauda equina syndrome.
- Often, the cauda equina syndrome may be incomplete, that is, some roots are spared or the syndrome is unilateral. This means that all features are not necessarily present but a potentially disabling disc prolapse may still have occurred. This implies that an index of suspicion is required in all patients with either urinary symptoms or saddle sensory symptoms, and this must be investigated urgently if symptoms are acute or progressive.

Principles of Acute Management

- MRI of the lumbosacral spine is the investigation of choice and should be obtained urgently when there are clinical features of cauda equina syndrome.
- If there is paraparesis or upper motor neuron signs, this is not consistent with cauda equina syndrome. Alternative pathology affecting spinal cord or brain must be considered and investigations planned accordingly.
- Where there is bladder involvement, a urinary catheter should be placed immediately as insensate urinary retention leads to stretching of the bladder and detrusor muscle which worsens function further.
- If MRI is unavailable or contraindicated but clinically required, consult neurosurgery. Consideration can be

given to transferring the patient for MRI or alternative investigation.

- If MRI excludes cauda equina compression, it is essential to examine the patient again and consider an alternative diagnosis. Are there upper motor neuron signs implying that the cervical or thoracic spinal cord is involved? It may be necessary to consult a neurologist.
- If disc prolapse is confirmed, referral to a neurosurgeon should be made urgently. Clinical features of duration and severity of the syndrome is key information for the referral. The patient can be transferred and offered urgent decompressive lumbar disc surgery with the aim of preventing further deterioration, relieving pain, and maximizing rehabilitation potential of bladder and bowel.

Discussion

Even following decompressive surgery, it is common for deficits to remain, and rehabilitation care is often necessary. In severe cauda equina syndrome, there is often permanent disability with incontinence of bladder and bowel, numbness, and loss of sexual function. Although it is as yet unproven whether surgery overnight offers any advantage over surgery on the next available list, it is widely accepted that once detected early decompression should be offered to minimize the resulting deficit.

Early diagnosis is therefore important but may sometimes be difficult owing to the fact that a potentially disabling disc prolapse may not produce all of the features of the cauda equina syndrome. There may also be difficulty if the patient cannot have MRI, for example, in cases of severe obesity, or if there are problems with availability of MRI. It is advisable that all patients with sensory symptoms affecting thighs or buttocks, or bilateral sensory symptoms, should be investigated for possible cauda equina compression. The diagnosis should also be considered for all patients with urinary retention or incontinence. In case of any difficulty, the case should be discussed with neurosurgery.

Key Points

1. Cauda equina syndrome involves the nerve roots in the lumbar spinal canal (*not* the spinal cord which ends at L1). As such, it is predominantly a syndrome of sensory changes and impaired continence. Motor deficits where they occur are of lower motor neuron type.
2. Painless urinary retention with overflow incontinence is a cardinal feature of severe cauda equina syndrome. A catheter should be placed early to prevent further stretching of the bladder.
3. If cauda equina syndrome is suspected, urgent MRI is necessary. If symptoms are acute or deteriorating, this may need to be obtained out of hours even if this requires the patient to be transferred.
4. Diagnostic difficulty may occur because the syndrome is often incomplete. If doubt arises and MRI is available, it is advisable to investigate. If MRI is not available, it is advisable to discuss the case with neurosurgery.
5. Cauda equina syndrome may result in severe permanent disability even where minimal motor deficit in the limbs exists because of impairment of continence and sexual function.

References

1. Patel H, Bouamra O, Woodford M, King A, Yates D, Lecky F, Trauma Audit and Research Network. Trends in head injury outcome from 1989 to 2003 and the effect of neurosurgical care: an observational study. Lancet. 2005;366:1538–44.

Index

I. Shergill et al. (eds.), *Surgical Emergencies in Clinical Practice*, 203
DOI 10.1007/978-1-4471-2876-2,
© Springer-Verlag London 2013

Printed by Printforce, the Netherlands